Mariem Nouira
Nadia Ben Mansour

Smoking epidemic among young Tunisians

Mariem Nouira
Nadia Ben Mansour

Smoking epidemic among young Tunisians

The scope and prospects for an effective fight against this scourge

ScienciaScripts

Imprint

Cover image: www.ingimage.com

This book is a translation from the original published under ISBN 978-620-6-72466-7.

Publisher:
Sciencia Scripts
is a trademark of
Dodo Books Indian Ocean Ltd. and OmniScriptum S.R.L publishing group

120 High Road, East Finchley, London, N2 9ED, United Kingdom
Str. Armeneasca 28/1, office 1, Chisinau MD-2012, Republic of Moldova, Europe
Printed at: see last page
ISBN: 978-620-8-32984-6

Contents

Resume

Smoking is a major public health issue worldwide.

The main objective of our work was to estimate the extent of smoking (cigarettes and cigarettes) among university students in Tunisia.

This was a cross-sectional descriptive online survey of students at the University of Tunis El Manar in 2022.

A total of 210 students were included in the study, with an average age of 21.5 years. The prevalence of Narguile use was 42.4% (CI95% [36.2 - 49.0]), with a significantly higher prevalence in men (p <10).$^{-3}$

More than a fifth (21.5%) thought that Narguile was less harmful than cigarettes and 21.2% had no intention of stopping smoking Narguile. The prevalence of cigarette smoking was 31.9% (95% CI [25.7 - 38.6]), with a significantly higher prevalence among men (P<0.01). The mean Fagerstrom score was 2.6 ± 2.2. The prevalence of smoking among young students was alarmingly high. Interventions to raise awareness and strengthen existing anti-smoking policies are a priority.

Tags: Tobacco consumption, Young adults, Attitude, Addiction

1 INTRODUCTION

Smoking is a major public health issue worldwide because of its high prevalence, its harmful effects on health and its heavy economic impact. According to the World Health Organisation (WHO), 1.3 billion people in the world smoke, with an estimated global prevalence of 22.3% in 2020. The majority of smokers, i.e. 80%, live in low- or middle-income countries [1]. Smoking is considered to be one of the leading causes of preventable death worldwide, responsible for more than 8 million deaths each year [2]. It is one of the main modifiable risk factors for non-communicable diseases, including cancers, chronic respiratory diseases and cardiovascular diseases [3].

Its frequency has increased alarmingly over the last two decades, especially in the Eastern Mediterranean region [4].

According to the World Health Organisation (WHO), 90 million adults in the region smoke [3].

The emergence of new trends in the use of Narguile has been observed mainly among young people, and in particular university students [5-7].

Indeed, the prevalence of Narguile use had exceeded 60% according to the results of a cross-sectional study conducted in 2016 on Narguile use among university students in the Eastern Mediterranean region [8]. This trend is partly explained by the social acceptability of smoking in all its forms and the influence of the media and social networks on young people [9].

The popularity of Narguile among young people is also due to the erroneous perception that it is less harmful than cigarettes, and the fact that the product comes in different flavours that are attractive to young people [10].

Tunisia is not immune to this serious scourge. According to the results of the national survey "Tunisian Health Examination Survey, 2016", around 25% of Tunisian adults use tobacco in various forms [11]. More than 13,200 Tunisians die each year from tobacco-related illnesses, accounting for 20% of all deaths in the country [12].

In Tunisia, according to the Global Youth Tobacco Surveys (GYTS), the prevalence of Narguile use among teenagers aged 13 to 15 rose from 5.8% in 2010 to 7.6% in 2017 [13]. This increase is even more worrying given the negative health impacts of Narguile, which are similar to those of cigarettes [14].

Although it has been shown that young adults represent the group most at risk of experimenting with (initiation to) and regularly consuming Narguile, few Tunisian studies have been interested in studying the use, attitudes and dependence of this population.

Thus, the main objective of this study was to estimate the prevalence of smoking in its two main forms, i.e. cigarette and Narguile use, among university students in Tunisia. Secondly, our objectives were to describe the degree of perception of harm and the intention to stop among users of these two forms of smoking. And also to determine the level of dependence and the factors associated with it.

2 METHODS

1. Type of study

This was a descriptive cross-sectional online survey of students at the University of Tunis El Manar. This study was conducted between July 2021 and January 2022. This work is part of a study that forms part of a multicentre research project between Lebanon and Tunisia to test the effectiveness of health warning labels specific to Narguile.

2. Study population

This study focused on a sample of students at the University of Tunis el Manar.

2.1. Inclusion criteria

All students aged between 18 and 34, resident in Tunisia (for at least 5 years), with an active e-mail address belonging to the University of Tunis El Manar, were included in the study.

2.2. Exclusion criteria

Students who refused to give informed consent before completing the questionnaire were excluded from the study.

3. Sample size

The minimum sample size was calculated using the following formula:

$$N= (Z_{a/2}^{2} \times p \times (l-p))/(i)^{2}$$

N: sample size

p: Expected frequency of Narguile use according to the results of the THES 2016 national survey, in which the prevalence of Narguile use among Tunisians aged 15 and over was 1.6%.

z: the critical value on the reduced centred normal distribution for a risk of error a (for a=5% z_a /2= 1.96)

i: degree of precision fixed at a 2%.

The minimum sample size calculated was 151 participants.

4. Data collection

This study was carried out exclusively online, given the epidemic situation relating to COVID 19, which prevented the collection of personal data in order to protect the safety of participants and investigators.

Participants were recruited using an e-mail distribution list of students at the University of Tunis El Manar. To increase the number of participants, another recruitment method was adopted in collaboration with the student association of the Faculty of Medicine of Tunis, Associa Med, by distributing leaflets to the students of the different faculties belonging to the University of Tunis El Manar with a brief description of the objectives and procedures of the study, as well as the contact details of the research team. Students interested in participating and who volunteered contacted the research team by telephone or e-mail so that they could take part in the study.

Subjects interested in taking part were invited to click on a link that redirected them to a questionnaire available via the Sphinx software and were asked to answer a few questions to confirm their eligibility.

Once eligible, participants were directed to the consent page. Only consenting participants were given access to the survey.

The questionnaire was available in two languages, Arabic and French, and participants were free to choose the language that suited them best.

The questionnaire (Appendix I) consisted of four parts

- **Part** 1: Socio-demographic data (age, gender, level of education and marital status (single, married, widowed or divorced)).
- **Part 2:** on the use of Narguile

- Frequency of use :

A current Narguile smoker was defined as one who smoked Narguile even less than once a month.

- Intention to initiate for non-smokers in the next 30 days
- The initiation age for smokers
- The intention to stop and reduce the use of Narguile within the next 30 days following the survey.
- Level of dependence on Narguile: assessed by The Syrian Center score

for Tobacco Studies-13 (SCTS-13) for the use of Narguile which comprised 13 items with three possible answers for each item: "False", "Somewhat true" or "True" with scores of 0, 1 or 2 respectively (score from 0 to 2/item). This score can vary from 0 to 26. The higher the score, the stronger the nicotine dependence [15].

- The extent to which people perceive Narguile to be harmful, comparing it with cigarettes and its serious effects on health.
- **Part 3:** Cigarette use :
- Frequency of use :

A current cigarette smoker was defined as someone who smoked cigarettes even less than once a month.

- Intention to initiate for non-smokers over the next year
- Intention to stop and reduce cigarette smoking
- Level of dependence: assessed by the Fagerstrom score [16]. This score is made up of 6 items: the time of the first cigarette smoked each day after waking up, abstention from smoking when it is forbidden, the cigarette that is most difficult to give up, the average number of cigarettes smoked per day, the frequency of smoking during the first hours of the day compared with the rest of the day, and smoking during illness. The score for each item may differ from one question to another. The Fagerstrom score ranges from 0 to 10. A subject can be classified into one of the following four categories according to the score results:
- Non-dependent: A score from 0 to 2
- Low dependency: A score of 3 to 4
- Moderately dependent: A score of 5 to 6
- Highly or very highly dependent: A score of 7 to 10
- The degree of perception of the serious health effects of cigarette smoking.
- **Part** 4: Other forms of tobacco consumption :

Frequency of current use of midwakh, cigars, flavoured cigars and electronic cigarettes.

5. Statistical analysis

For descriptive statistics, qualitative variables were expressed in terms of absolute and relative frequencies (percentages), while quantitative variables were expressed in terms of mean (± standard deviation).

The chi-square test was used to compare the percentages between the different groups.

Multiple linear regression was used to study the factors associated with the total dependence score on Narguile SCTS-13. A p-value < 0.05 was considered significant for all statistical tests used. Statistical analysis was performed using SPSS software (version 23.0, IBM Corp).

6. Bibliographic research

We used Zotero for bibliographic management.

The databases consulted during the bibliographic search were : Pubmed, Scopus, Google Scholar and Science direct.

We used the following keywords: young adult, university students, tobacco smoking, water-pipe smoking. The research was also conducted in English using the following keywords: young adult, university students, tobacco smoking, water-pipe smoking.

Our bibliographic research also included sites and reports from international organisations such as the World Health Organisation, as well as reports from Tunisian national surveys on smoking (Global Youth Tobacco survey, MED SPAD, and Tunisian Health Examination Survey).

7. Ethical considerations

All participants were informed of the framework and main purpose of the study prior to their participation and were cordially invited to y participate based on their own volition.

All this information was mentioned in the text of the email.

All data collected and analysed was treated anonymously. Data confidentiality was respected during and after data collection. All information collected was stored in a secure location and used for research purposes only. The approval of the Ethics Committee of the Faculty of Medicine of Tunis was obtained before the study was carried out, with the approval number CE-FMT/2019/05/FMT/V1.

3 RESULTS

1. Description of the study population

A total of 210 students were included in the study.

The socio-demographic characteristics of the study population are shown in Table I.

1.1 Age distribution

The mean age was 21.5 ± 2.3 years, with extremes ranging from 18 to 34 years (Figure 1). The majority of participants (85.2%) were aged between 18 and 23 years (Table I).

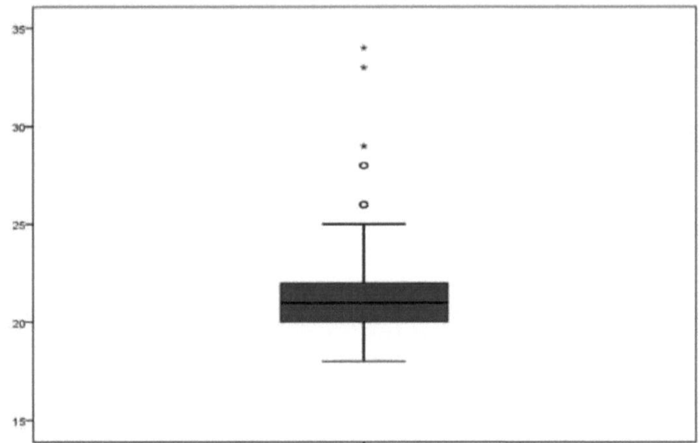

Figure 1: Box plot of participants' ages

1.2 Breakdown by gender

The study population consisted of 129 women (61.4%) and 81 men (38.6%), with a sex ratio (male/female) of 0.63 (Table I).

1.3 Breakdown by level of education

More than half (61.5%) of the students were in 2nd cycle university (table I).

1.4 Breakdown by marital status

The majority of students (n=203 or 98.1%) were single (table I).

Table I: Distribution of students by socio-demographic characteristics demographic characteristics (gender, age groups, marital status and level of level of education)

Socio-demographic characteristics	Number of employees (%)
Sex	
Male	81 (38,6)
Female	129 (61,4)
Age groups (years)	
[18-20]	80 (38,1)
[21-23]	99 (47,1)
>24	31 (14,8)
Level of education *	
Ier university cycle	70 (38,5)
2ème university cycle	112 (61,5)
Marital status *	
Single	203 (98,1)
Marie/couple	3 (1,4)
Divorce/separation	1 (0,5)

* *missing data*

2. Use of Narguile

2.1 Prevalence of Narguile use

A total of 89 of the 210 students were current Narguile smokers, a prevalence of 42.4% (1Cэ5% [36.2 - 49.0]). The frequency of exclusive Narguile smoking (not associated with cigarettes) was 18.1% (n=38) with CI95% [13.5 - 23.9], while 51 were smokers of Narguile and cigarettes at the same time, i.e. a prevalence of 24.3% (CI95% [19.0 - 30.5]). Of the smokers responding to the question on the frequency of Narguile use (n= 79), most (79.7%) smoked Narguile less than once a month, while 5.1% smoked Narguile daily or at least once a week (Figure 2).

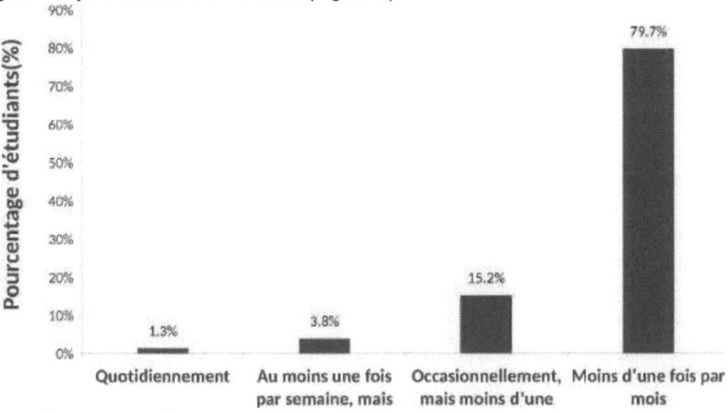

Figure 2: Breakdown of current Narguile smokers by frequency of consumption (N=79)

The average age of Narguile's initiation was 17.8, with extremes ranging from 10 to 24. The average duration of use of Narguile was 3.8 ± 2.3 years, with a maximum of 11 years.

Of the 210 students, 118 had never smoked Narguile, a prevalence of 56.2% (IC95% [49.0 - 62.9]).

Only three said they used to smoke Narguile but had stopped.

Among the current Narguile non-smokers who responded to the question (n=114), the main reasons given for not smoking Narguile were the fact of being at the centre of all types of smoking (n=64; 56.1%) and the fact of thinking that it is bad for health (n=41; 36.0%) (Figure 3).

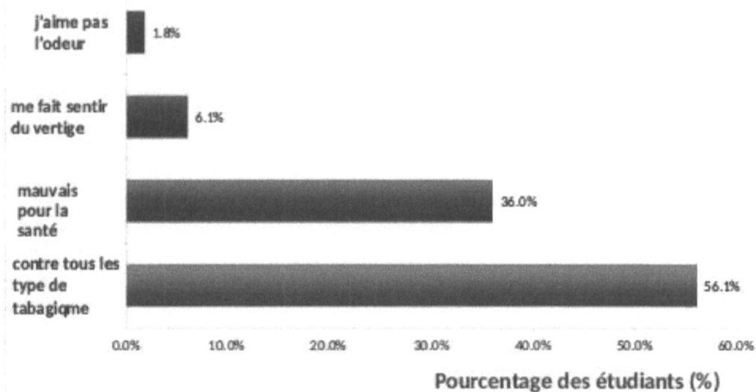

Figure 3 : Reasons given for not smoking Narguile (N= 114)

2.2 Frequency of Narguile use by socio-demographic characteristics

Table II shows the results of the study of the association between current Narguile smoking and never having used Narguile, with the socio-demographic characteristics of the students.

2.2.1 Use of Narguile by gender

Male sex was significantly associated with Narguile use (60.5% in men vs. 31.0% in women; OR=3.4; $p < 10^{'3}$). The frequency of women who had never smoked Narguile was significantly higher than that of men ($p < 10^{'3}$), (table II).

2.2.2 Use of Narguile by age group

There was no significant difference in Narguile use between the different age groups (46.3% of smokers aged [18 to 20] vs. 43.4% of smokers aged [21 to 23] vs. 29.0% of smokers aged 24 or over; p=0.2). The frequency of never having smoked Narguile was not significantly associated with age (p=0.1) (table II).

2.2.3 Use of Narguile according to marital status

There was no significant difference in Narguile use between single students and students with another marital status (42.4% smokers among single students vs. 25.0% smokers among other students, p=0.6). The frequency of never having smoked Narguile was not as significantly associated with marital status (p=0.6), (table II).

2.2.4 Use of Narguile by level of education

There was no significant difference in Narguile use between undergraduate and postgraduate students (44.3% undergraduate vs. 39.3% postgraduate, p=0.5). The frequency of never having smoked Narguile was not significantly associated with the level of education (p=0.5) (Table II).

Table II: Study of socio-demographic factors associated with Narguile use status (current smoker versus never smoker)

Status of Narguile use								
	Current smoker (N=89)				**Never used (N=118)**			
Student characteristics	**N**	**% (lines)**	OR	**Value of p**	**N**	**% (lines)**	OR	**Value of p**
Gender				**$<10^{-3}$**				**$<10^{-3}$**
Men	49	60,5	3,4 [1,9-6,1]		31	38,3	ref	
Women	40	31,0	ref		87	67,4	3,3 [1.9-5.9]	
Age groups (years)				0,2				0,1
[18-20]	37	46,3	-		42	52,5	-	
[21-23]	43	43,4			54	54,5		
> 24	9	29,0			22	71,0		
Marital status *				0,6				0,6

Single	86	42,4	-		114	56,2	-	
Other	1	25,0			3	75,0		
Level of education*				0,5				0,5
Ier cycle	31	44,3	-		38	54,3	-	
2®me cycle	44	39,3			66	58,9		

* : missing data ; .ref: reference category

2.3 Dependency on Narguile

Of the 75 current Narguile smokers who responded, 10.7% had Narguile at home and 13.3% usually prepared their own Narguile for smoking.

2.3.1 Degree of dependence perceived by Narguile smokers

Among 72 current Narguile smokers, 94.4% felt that they were not addicted to Narguile and 2.8% felt that they were very addicted to Narguile (Figure 4).

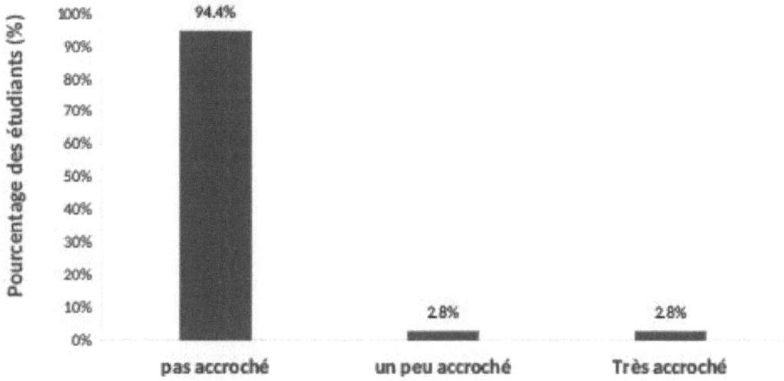

Figure 4: Degree of dependence on Narguile perceived by smokers (N=72).

2.3.2 Degree of dependence assessed by The Syrian Center for Tobacco Studies-13 (SCTS-13) score

The mean Narguile dependence score was 6.7 ± 5.0 with extremes ranging from 0 to 26. The interquartile range of the score was [2 - 10], indicating that 75% of Narguile smokers had a score < 10 (Figure 5).

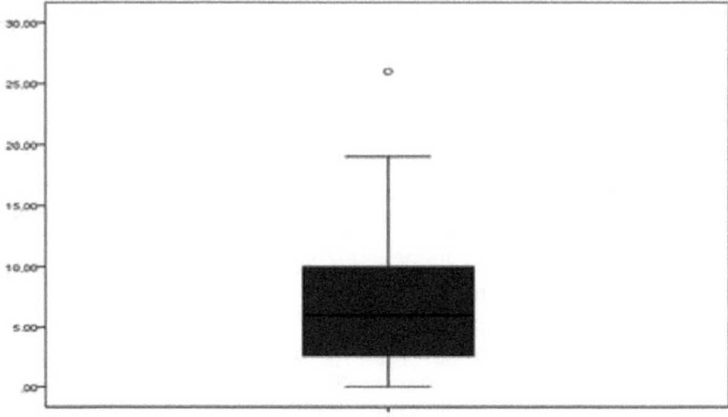

Figure 5: Box plot of the Narguile SCTS-13 dependency score

The responses of 75 Narguile smokers to the 13 items making up the SCTS-13 Narguile Dependence Score are detailed in Table III.

Table III: Distribution of responses from Narguile smokers according to the different items in the Narguile dependence score (SCTS-13), (N=75)

Items SCTS-13	NO N (%)	SOMEWHAT TRUE N (%)	TRUE N (%)
Item 1 (SCTS-1)			
Most of my friends smoke Narguile	**21** **(28,0)**	**36** **(48,0)**	**18** **(24,0)**
Item 2 (SCTS-2)			
Just the sight or smell of Narguile is enough for me make you want to smoke	**34** **(45,3)**	**26** **(34,7)**	**15** **(20,0)**
Item 3 (SCTS-3)			
Even if I was sure that Narguile was no good for my health, I'd still smoke just as often	**50** **(66,7)**	**21** **(28,0)**	**04** **(5,3)**
Item 4 (SCTS-4)			
Smoking a Narguile makes me happy	**35** **(46,7)**	**34** **(45,3)**	**06** **(8,0)**
Item 5 (SCTS-5)			
Smoking a Narguile makes me feel full of energy	**48** **(64,0)**	**25** **(33,3)**	**02** **(2,7)**
Item 6 (SCTS-6)			
If the cost of Narguile doubled, I'd still smoke as often	**55** **(73,3)**	**17** **(22,7)**	**03** **(4,0)**
Item 7 (SCTS-7)			
When I smoke Narguile, I feel less sad or depressed	**48** **(64,0)**	**25** **(33,3)**	**02** **(2,7)**
Item 8 (SCTS-8)			
It would be very difficult for me to be in a situation like that. restaurant and not to smoke the Narguile	**60** **(80,0)**	**13** **(17,3)**	**02** **(2,7)**
Item 9 (SCTS-9)			
Smoking a Narguile is a good way to help me reward	**54** **(72,0)**	**12** **(16,0)**	**09** **(12,0)**
Item 10 (SCTS-10)			
It would be difficult for me to refuse an invitation to smoke a Narguile	**39** **(52,0)**	**24** **(32,0)**	**12** **(16,0)**
Item 11 (SCTS-11)			
I usually smoke Narguile with friends or in cafés / restaurants	**25** **(33,3)**	**25** **(33,3)**	**25** **(33,3)**
Item 12 (SCTS-12)			
If my Narguile smoking session were to be interrupted, I would be upset	**57** **(76,0)**	**15** **(20,0)**	**03** **(4,0)**
Item 13 (SCTS-13)			
When I smoke a water pipe, I feel less irritable, frustrated or angry	**50** **(66,7)**	**21** **(28,0)**	**04** **(5,3)**

The factors that were significantly associated with a higher SCTS-13 Narguile dependence score, following simple linear regression, were the fact of having a Narguile at home, the fact of preparing one's own Narguile and the fact of being a Narguile and cigarette smoker at the same time (Table IV).

Table IV: Results of simple linear regression to study the factors associated with the total dependence score on Narguile SCTS-13

	Total score SCTS-13 Regression coefficient Crude P	P
Gender		0,8

Women	+ 0,229	
Men	ref	
Age groups		0,5
> 24	+ 0,56	
[21-23]	+ 1,24	
[18-20]	ref	
Level of education		0,4
2ème cycle	-1,02	
Ier cycle	ref	
Frequency of use of Narguile		0,17
Less than once a month	+ 0,18	
Occasionally, but less than once a week	+ 3,85	
At least once a week, but not every day	+ 3,33	
Daily	ref	
Having a Narguile at home		**0,03**
Yes	+ 3,95	
No	.ref	
Making your own Narguile		**0,005**
Yes	+ *4,70*	
No	ref	
Age of initiation for Turner the Narguile	0,01	0,9
Duration of use of Narguile	+ 0,07	0,7
Smoking Narguile and cigarettes at the same time		**0,008**
Yes	+ 3,24	
No	ref	
Degree of perceived addiction to Narguile (compared to cigarettes)		0,16
Less addictive	+ 1,74	
Other answer *("Equally addictive"; "more addictive"; "I don't know")*	ref	
Degree of perceived harmfulness of Narguile (compared with cigarettes)		0,24
Less harmful	+ 1,92	
Other answer *("Equally harmful"; "more harmful"; "I don't know")*	ref	
Degree of perception of serious health effects of Narguile		0,8
Not at all	+ 0,45	
Other answer *((From "a little" to "a lot")*	ref	
Perception of the degree to which life is affected by health problems linked to the use of Narguile		0,3
Not at all	-2,27	
Other answer *((From "a little" to "a lot")*	ref	

ref: cak'gorie de rdfdrence

The factors independently associated with a higher SCTS-13 total score for dependence on Narguile (following multiple linear regression) were the fact of preparing one's own Narguile (0 = + 4.05; p=0.04), and the fact of smoking Narguile and cigarettes at the same time (0 = + 3.13; p=0.01) (Table V).

Table V: Results of the final multiple linear regression model to study the factors independently associated with the total dependence score on Narguile SCTS-13

	Total score SCTS-13 Adjusted regression coefficient p	P
Usually prepare its own Narguile		0,04
Yes	+ 4,05	
No	ref	
Smoking Narguile and cigarettes at the same time		0,01
Yes	+ 3,13	
No	ref	

ref: *rdfdrence category*

2.4 Frequency of Narguile smokers who have previously tried to stop using Narguile

Among 75 Narguile smokers, 33 (44%) had tried to stop using Narguile before. There was no significant difference by sex (42.9% of men had tried to quit vs. 45.5% of women; p= 0.8). The fact of having tried to stop using Narguile was not significantly associated with the degree of perceived harmfulness (p= 0.7) and serious health effects (p= 0.7) of Narguile use compared with cigarettes. Similarly, the perceived degree to which Narguile use affected smokers' lives was not significantly associated with the fact of having tried to stop using Narguile (p=0.6).

2.5 Students' attitudes towards the use of Narguile

The results of the comparison of students' attitudes to Narguile use according to smoking and non-smoking status are shown in Table VI.

2.5.1 Perception of Narguile addiction

Of the 194 students, smokers and non-smokers of Narguile, who answered the question comparing the degree of perceived addiction due to Narguile compared to cigarettes, 28.4% thought that Narguile use is less addictive than cigarettes and 25.7% did not know how to answer the question. Whereas 45.9% thought it was equally or even more addictive than cigarettes (Figure 6). There was no significant difference when comparing the responses of current Narguile smokers and non-smokers (33.3% of current Narguile smokers thought that Narguile is less addictive than cigarettes vs. 25.2% of Narguile non-smokers; p=0.2), (Table VI).

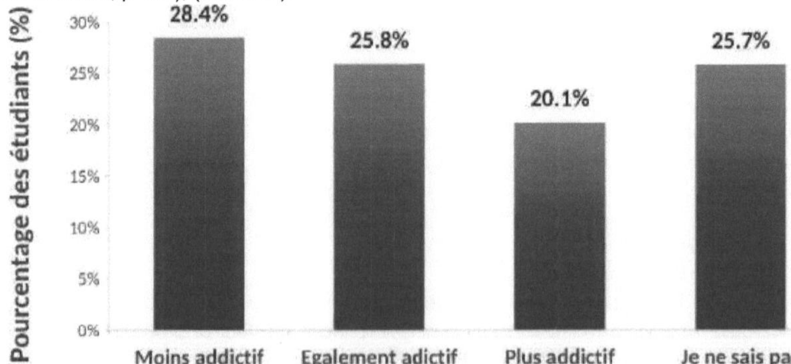

Figure 6: Degree of perceived addiction to Narguile compared with cigarettes among all students (N=194).

2.5.2 Perception of the harm done to Narguile's health

Of the 196 students, smokers and non-smokers of Narguile, who answered the question comparing the degree of harmfulness of Narguile to cigarettes, 8.7% thought that Narguile use was less harmful than cigarettes and 12.8% did not know how to answer the question. Whereas 78.6% thought it was equally or even more harmful than cigarettes (Figure 7). The frequency of Narguile smokers who thought that Narguile is less harmful to health than cigarettes was significantly higher than that of Narguile non-smokers (14.7% of smokers vs. 5.0% of Narguile non-smokers; p=0.01), (Table VI).

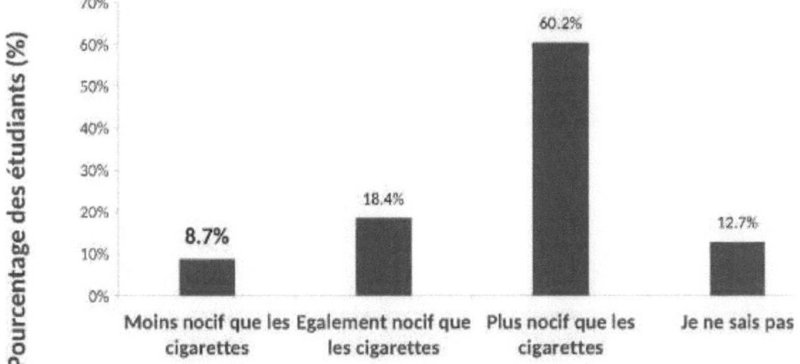

Figure 7: Degree of perceived harmfulness of Narguile compared with cigarettes among all students (N=196)

2.5.3 Degree of perception of serious health effects of Narguile

Of the 210 students, smokers and non-smokers of Narguile, who answered the question measuring the degree of perception of the serious health effects of Narguile, 8.6% thought that Narguile use had no serious health effects at all, and 12.9% thought that it had few serious effects (Figure 8). There was no significant difference when comparing the responses of current Narguile smokers and non-smokers (11.2% of current Narguile smokers thought that Narguile has no serious health effects at all vs. 6.6% of Narguile non-smokers; p=0.2), (Table V).

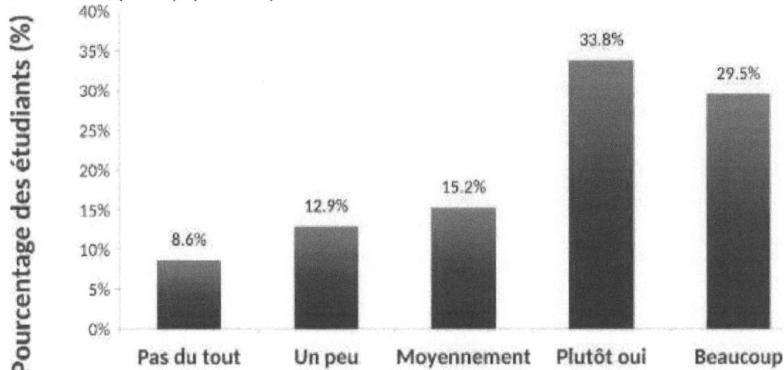

Figure 8: Degree of perception of the serious health effects of Narguile among Narguile smokers and non-smokers (N=210)

2.5.4 Perception of the degree to which life is affected by health problems linked

to the use of Narguile

Among the 210 students, smokers and non-smokers of Narguile, who answered the question measuring the perceived degree to which health problems related to Narguile use affect their lives, 7.1% thought that health problems related to Narguile use do not affect smokers' lives at all, and 9.5% thought that they affect smokers' lives to a small extent (Figure 9). There was no significant difference when comparing the responses of current Narguile smokers and non-smokers (7.9% of current Narguile smokers thought that Narguile does not affect smokers' lives at all vs. 6.6% of Narguile non-smokers; p=0.7), (Table VI).

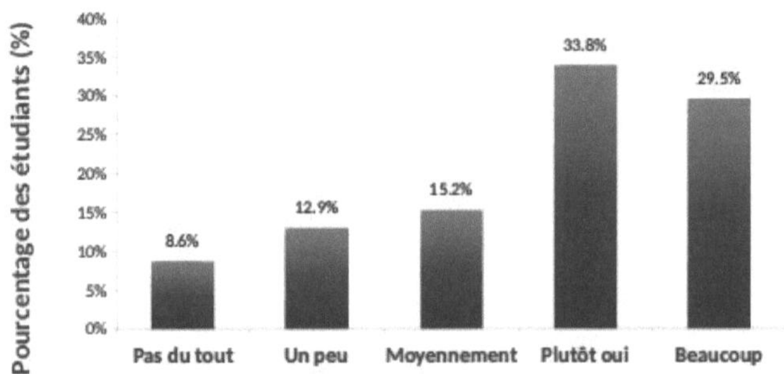

Figure 9: Perceived degree to which life is affected by Narguile-related health problems among smokers and non-smokers in Narguile (№210)

Table VI: Comparison of students' attitudes to Narguile use according to smoking and non-smoking status

	Students' attitudes towards the use of Narguile		**P**
	Degree of perceived **addiction** to Narguile compared to cigarettes (N= 194)		
Use of Narguile	**Less addictive N (% line)**	**Other answer N (% line)**	0,2
Smoker	25 (33,3)	50 (66,7)	
Non-smoking	30 (25,2)	89 (74,8)	
	Perceived degree **of harm done** to health by Narguile compared with cigarettes (N= 196)		**0,01**
Use of Narguile	**Less harmful N (% line)**	**Other answer N (% line)**	
Smoker	11 (14,7)	64 (85,3)	
Non-smoking	06 (5,0)	115 (95,0)	
	Degree of perception of **serious** health **effects** of Narguile (N= 210)		0,2
Use of Narguile	**Not at all N (% line)**	**Other answer N (% line)**	
Smoker	10 (11,2)	79 (88,8)	
Non-smoking	08 (6,6)	113 (93,4)	
	Perceived degree to which health problems linked to Narguile use **affect life** (N= 210)		0,7
Use of Narguile	**Not at all N (% line)**	**Other answer N (% line)**	

Smoker	07 (7,9)	82 (92,1)
Non-smoking	08 (6,6)	113 (93,4)

2.5.5 Intention to initiate use of Narguile

Of the current Narguile non-smokers who answered the question (n=89) about their intention to start using Narguile in the next 30 days, 77.6% had no such intention at all. Whereas 20 students (22.4%) intended to start using Narguile in the near future, with an intensity ranging from "a little" to "a lot" (Figure 10). The intention to initiate Narguile use was not significantly different between men and women (23.1% of women intended to initiate Narguile vs. 20.8% of men; p= 0.8). There was no significant association between age (p=0.7), marital status (p=l.0), level of university education (p=0.6), being a cigarette smoker (p= 1.0) and intention to initiate Narguile use. Similarly, there was no significant association between the degree of perceived harmfulness (p=0.5), and serious health effects (p=0.6) of Narguile use and the intention to initiate its use (Table MI).

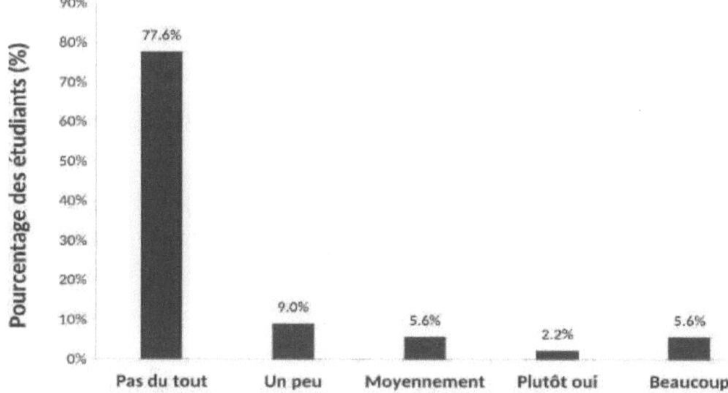

Figure 10 : Intention d'initier l'usage de Narguilé parmi les non-fumeurs (N=89)

Table VII: Study of factors associated with intention to initiate Narguile use in Narguile non-smokers

	Intention to initiate the use of Narguile		
Features	**YES N(% line)**	**NO N(% line)**	**P**
Gender			0,8
Men	5 (20,8)	19 (79,2)	
Woman	15 (23,1)	50 (76,9)	
Age groups (years)			0,7
[18-23]	17 (23,6)	55 (76,4)	
>24	3 (17,6)	14 (82,4)	
Marital status			1,0
Single	19 (22,4)	66 (77,6)	
Other status **(Marie, couple, divorce)**	0 (0,0)	3 (100,0)	
Level of university education			0,6
1st cycle	6 (23,1)	20 (76,9)	

2nd cycle	9 (18,4)	40 (81,6)	
Smoking (cigarettes)			1,0
Yes	2 (18,2)	9 (81,8)	
No	18 (23,1)	60 (76,9)	
Иедгё of perceived addiction due to Narguite use (comparing it to cigarettes)			0,5
Less addictive than cigarettes.	3 (13,6)	19 (86,4)	
Other answer *("Equally addictive"; "more addictive"; "I don't know")*	15 (23,1)	50 (76,9)	
Иедгё of perceived harmfulness of Narguite (comparing it to cigarettes)			0,5
Less harmful than the cigarettes	1 (33,3)	2 (66,7)	
Other answer *("Equally harmful"; "more harmful"; "I don't know")*	19 (22,1)	67 (77,9)	
Иедгё of perception of serious health effects of Narguite.			0,6
Not at all	2 (33,3)	4 (66,7)	
Other answer *((Ranging from "a little" to "a lot")*	18 (21,7)	65 (78,3)	
Perception of дедгё of life affectation by healthproblems Hё$ a Pusage de Narguite			0,6
Not at all	2 (33,3)	4 (66,7)	
Other answer *(Ranging from "a little" to "a lot")*	18 (21,7)	65 (78,3)	
Other smokers encourage you to smoke Narguile			0,5
Yes	6 (25,0)	18 (75,0)	
No	12 (19,4)	50 (80,6)	0,8
Accompanying friends/family on outings to smoke Narguite			
Yes	10 (21,7)	36 (78,3)	
No	8 (20,0)	32 (80,0)	0,5

Number of people in the family who smoke Narguile			
At least 1 member	6 (26,1)	17 (73,9)	
No member	12 (19,0)	51 (81,0)	
Number of friends who smoke Narguile			0,4
At least 1 friend	10 (17,9)	46 (82,1)	
No friends	8 (26,7)	22 (73,3)	

2.5.6 The intention to stop using Narguile

Of the 66 current Narguile smokers who answered the question, 21.2% did not intend to stop smoking Narguile at all. Only 19.7% intended to stop using Narguile "a lot" (Figure 11). The intention to stop using Narguile was significantly associated with age (84.2% of Narguile smokers aged [18-23] years intended to stop vs. 44.4% aged > 24 years; p=0.01), university education (95.5% of Narguile smokers enrolled in undergraduate studies intended to stop vs. 62.5% enrolled in postgraduate studies; p=0.005). However, the intention to stop using Narguile was not significantly associated with the duration of Narguile use (p=0.8), nor with the total Narguile dependence score (SCTS-13) (p=0.9)

.

Furthermore, the intention to stop using Narguile among smokers who thought that Narguile use had no serious health effects at all was significantly lower (33.3%) than that of Narguile smokers who thought the opposite (83.3%; p=0.01). Similarly, the intention to stop using Narguile among smokers who thought that health problems linked to Narguile use did not affect a smoker's life at all, was significantly lower (25.0%) than that of Narguile smokers who thought the opposite (82.3%); p=0.02). Furthermore, the fact of having tried to stop using Narguile was not significantly associated with the intention to stop using Narguile (86.4% of those who had already tried to stop using Narguile intended to stop, compared with 75% of those who had not tried to stop; p=0.4), (Table VIII).

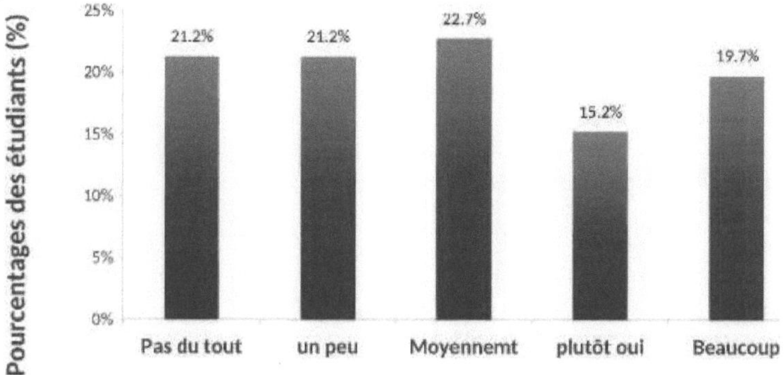

Figure 11: Intention to stop using Narguile among current smokers **(N=66)**

Table VIII: Study of factors associated with the intention to stop using Narguile among current Narguile smokers

	Intention to stop using Narguile		
Features	**YES**	**NO N (% line)**	**P**

	N (% line)			
Gender			0,5	
Men	29 (76,3)	9 (23,7)		
Woman	23 (82,1)	5 (17,9)		**0,01**
Age groups (years)				
[18-23]	48 (84,2)	9 (15,8)		
>24	4 (44,4)	5 (55,6)		
Marital status			1,0	
Single	50 (78,1)	14 (21,9)		
Other status **(Marie, couple, divorce)**	1 (100,0)	0 (0,0)		
Level of university education				**0,005**
1st cycle	21 (95,5)	1 (4,5)		
2nd cycle	20 (62,5)	12 (37,5)		
Иuгёе use of Narguile (in annties)			0,8	
Median [IQR]*	3,0 [2,0-6,0]	3,5 [2,75-4,25]		
Total dependency score for Narguile (SCTS-13)			0,9	
Median [IQR]*	6,0 [2,0-11,0]	6,0 [4,0-10,0]		
Smoking (cigarettes)			0,8	
Yes	28 (77,8)	8 (22,2)		
No	24 (80,0)	6 (20,0)	0,7	
Иеdгё perception of addiction due to Narguite use (comparing it to cigarettes)				
Less addictive than cigarettes	15 (83,3)	3 (16,7)		
Other answer *("Equallyaddictive"; "more addictive"; "I don't know")*	28 (77,8)	8 (22,2)		
Иеdгё of perceived harmfulness of Narguite (in comparing it to cigarettes)			0,4	
Less harmful than cigarettes	7 (70,0)	3 (30,0)		
Other answer *("Equally harmful"; "more harmful"; "I don't know")*	36 (81,8)	8 (18,2)		**0,01**
Иеdгё of perception of serious health effects of Narguite				
Not at all.	2 (33,3)	4 (66,7)		
Other answer *(*	50 (83,3)	10 (16,7)		

"a little' until "many")			**0,02**
Perception of the degree to which life is affected by health problems* related *to drug use Narguite			
Not at all	1 (25,0)	3 (75,0)	
Other answer *(Ranging from "a little" to "a lot")*	51 (82,3)	11 (17,7)	
Have eззayë to stop using			0,4
Narguite Yes	19 (86,4)	3 (13,6)	
No	24 (75,0)	8 (25,0)	

*IQR]: Interquartile range

As for the degree of motivation to stop using Narguile in the next 30 days, 19.7% (out of 66 respondents) were not at all motivated, compared with a majority of 80.3% who were motivated, with degrees ranging from "a little" to "a lot" (Figure 12).

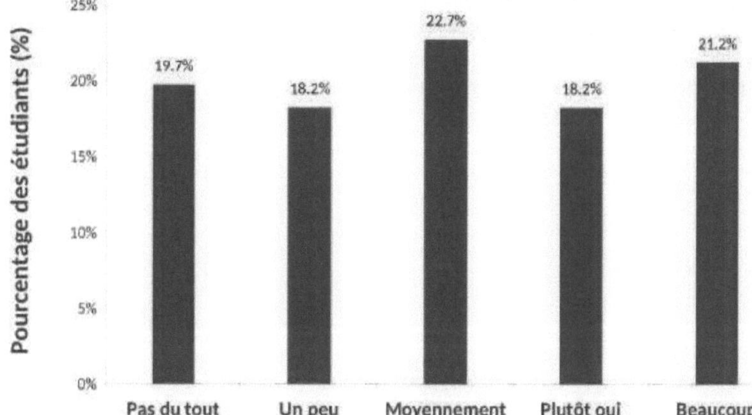

Figure 12: Level of motivation to stop using Narguile in the next 30 days among current smokers (N=66)

2.5.7 The intention to reduce the frequency of use of Narguile :

Of the 66 current Narguile smokers who answered the question, 21.2% had no intention at all of reducing the frequency of Narguile use in the next 30 days. Whereas 78.8% had this intention, with degrees ranging from "a little" to "a lot" (Figure 13).

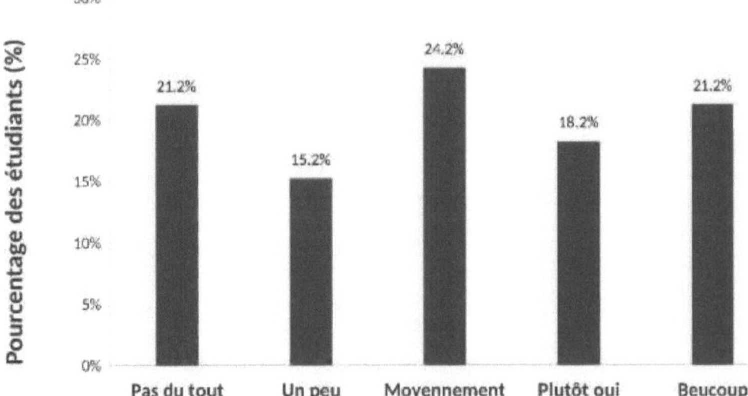

Figure 13: Intention to reduce frequency of Narguile use in the next 30 days among current smokers (N=66)

3. Cigarette smoking

3.1 Prevalence of cigarette smoking

A total of 67 of the 210 participants reported being current cigarette smokers, representing a prevalence of 31.9% (IC95% [25.7 - 38.6]). Of these, 37 (55.2%) smoked daily (Figure 14). The frequency of exclusive cigarette smoking (not associated with Narguile) was 7.6% (n=16) with 95% CI [4.7 - 12.0].

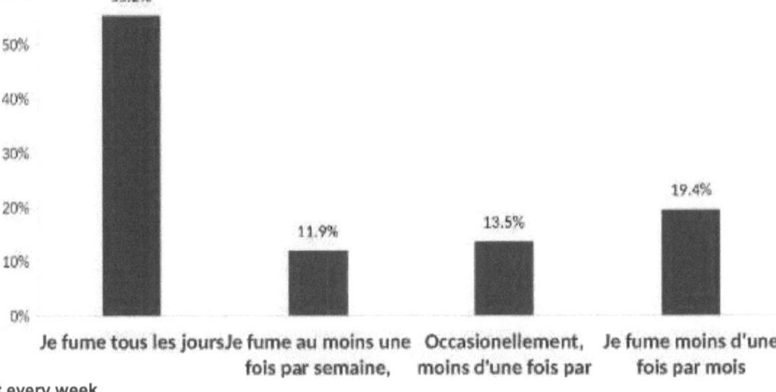

Figure 14: Breakdown of current cigarette smokers by frequency of consumption consumption (N=67)

Of the 210 participants, 131 said they had never smoked cigarettes, representing a prevalence of 62.4% (IC95% [56.2 - 68.6]).

Twelve students, or 5.7% (95% CI [2.9 - 9.0]), said they used to smoke cigarettes but had stopped.

3.2 Frequency of cigarette smoking by socio-demographic characteristics :

Table IX shows the results of the study of the association between current cigarette smoking and the fact of never having smoked cigarettes, with the socio-demographic characteristics of the students.

The factors significantly associated with cigarette smoking were sex (p= 0.002) and age (p=0.02) (table IX).

3.2.1 Cigarette smoking by sex

Male sex was significantly associated with cigarette use (44.4% in men vs. 24.0% in women; OR=2.5; p= 0.002). The frequency of women having never smoked cigarettes was significantly higher than that of men (OR= 3.2; p <10'^{3}), (table IX).

3.2.2 Cigarette smoking by age group

There was a significant difference in cigarette smoking by age group (30.0% of smokers aged [18 to 20] vs. 39.4% of smokers aged [21 to 23] vs. 12.9% of smokers aged 24 or more; p=0.02). The frequency of never having smoked cigarettes was significantly higher among students aged >24 years (OR=2.9 [1.02-8.5]; p=0.01), (table IX).

3.2.3 Cigarette smoking by marital status

There was no significant difference in cigarette use between single students and students with another marital status (p=0.3). Never having smoked cigarettes was also not significantly associated with marital status (p=0.3), (table IX).

3.2.4 Cigarette smoking by level of education

There was no significant difference in cigarette use between undergraduates and postgraduates (27.1% undergraduates vs. 32.1% postgraduates, p=0.5). The fact of never having smoked cigarettes was not significantly associated with the level of education (p=0.8), (table IX).

Table IX: Study of socio-demographic factors associated with cigarette smoking status (current smoker versus never smoker)

Cigarette smoking status							
Current smoker (N= 67) Never used (N=131)							
Features		**N%ORPN%ORP**					
of students	**(lines)**	**(lines)**					
Gender	**0,002**	**<IO-^{3}**					
Men	3644	,	42,5 [1.4-4.5]		3745	,7	.ref
Women	3124.0	.	ref9472 .		93.2 [l.8-5.7]		
Age groups	**0,**	**020,01**					
(years)							
[18-20]	2430.	02.9 [0.9-9.2]		5163	.8	.ref	
[21-23]	3939,	44,4 [1,4-13,5]		5454	,	50,7 [0.4-1.3]	
> 24	412	.9 .	ref2683 .		92.9 [1.02-8.5]		
Status	0,	30,3					
matrimonial *							
Single	6632,	5-12561 ,		6	-		
Other		**00, 04100**					
Level	**0,**	**50,8**					
of studies*							
Ier cycle	1927,	1-4564 ,		3-			
2eme cycle	3632,	17062 ,5					

** : missing data ; .ref: reference category*

3.3 Cigarette addiction according to the Fagerstrom score

Among the current cigarette smokers (N=67) who responded to the Fagerstrom dependence score, 6 students (9.0%) declared that they smoked their first cigarette within the first 5 minutes after waking up; 14 (20.9%) found it difficult to refrain from smoking in places where it is forbidden; 47 (70.1%) had the most difficulty giving up their first cigarette in the morning; 7 (10.5%) smoked 21 or more cigarettes on average per day; 14 (20.9%) smoked at a faster rate in the morning than during the rest of the day and 19 (28.4%) smoked even when they were ill (to the point of having to stay in bed for most of the day), (Table X).

Table X: Breakdown of responses from current cigarette smokers according to the different items in the Fagerstrom dependency score, (N=67)

Fagerstrom score				
FAGERSTROM 1 How soon after waking up do you smoke your first cigarette?	**Within 5 first minutes N (%)** 6 (9.0)	**Between 6 and 30 minutes N (%)** 10 (14,9)	**Between 31 and 60 minutes N (%)** 10 (14,9)	**More than 60 minutes N (%)** 41 (61,2)
FAGERSTROM 2 Do you find it difficult to refrain from smoking in places where it is prohibited?	**YES** 14 (20,9)		**NO** 53 (79,1)	
FAGERSTROM 3 Which cigarette of the day would you find hardest to give up?	**First thing in the morning** 47 (70,1)		**Any other** 20 (29,9)	
FAGERSTROM 4 How many cigarettes do you smoke per day on average?	**31 or more** 1 (1,5)	**21a30** 6 (9,0)	**lla20** 18 (26,9)	**10 or less** 42 (62,7)
FAGERSTROM 5 Do you smoke at closer intervals in the early hours of the morning than during the rest of the day?	**YES** 14 (20,9)		**NO** 53 (79,1)	
FAGERSTROM 6 Do you smoke when you're ill, to the extent that you have to stay in bed most of the day?	**YES** 19 (28,4)		**NO** 48 (71,6)	

The mean Fagerstrom score was 2.6 ± 2.2 with extremes ranging from 0 to 10. The interquartile range of the score was [1 - 4], indicating that 75% of cigarette smokers had a score < 4 (Figure 15).

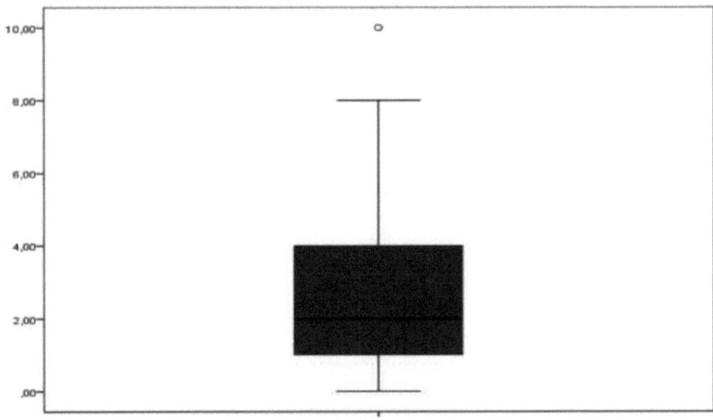

Figure 15: Box plot of the Fagerstrom score

In total, 27 cigarette-smoking students (40.3%) were dependent on Nicotine, with a level of dependence ranging from "Weakly" to "Strongly" dependent. Of all the students who smoked cigarettes (N=67), 5 were heavily dependent (7.5%) (Figure 16).

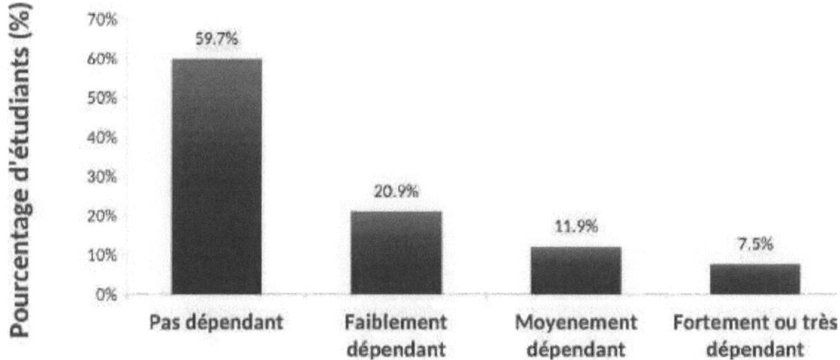

Figure 16: Distribution of current cigarette smokers according to their level of nicotine dependence, based on the Fagerstrom score (N=67)

The factors significantly associated with nicotine dependence among current cigarette smokers according to the Fagerstrom score were male sex (OR= 4.3 [1.5-12.5]; p= 0.006), age > 24 years (OR= 2.7 [1.9-3.8]; p= 0.02), the fact of smoking an electronic cigarette and a traditional cigarette at the same time (OR= 7.3 [1.9-28.9]; p= 0.03) and the fact of smoking other forms of smoking (such as cigars, *Midwakh* or flavoured cigars) and a traditional cigarette at the same time (OR= 3.3 [1.02-10.3]; p= 0.04), (Table XI).

Table XI: Study of factors associated with Nicotine dependence in the current cigarette smokers by Fagerstrom score (N=67)

	Nicotine dependence according to Fagerstrom score			
Features	**YES** *("Low" to "Strongly" dependent)* **N(% line)**	**NO** **N (% line)**	**OR [IC95%]**	**P**
Gender				**0,006**
Men	20 (55,6)	16 (44,4)	4,3 [1,5-12,5]	
Woman	07 (22,6)	24 (77,4)	.ref	
Age groups (years)				**0,02**
[18-23]	23 (36,5)	40 (63,5)	.ref	
>24	04 (100,0)	0 (0,0)	2,7 [l,9-3,8]	
Marital status*				
Single	27 (40,9)	39 (59,1)		
Other status **(Marie, couple, divorce)**	0 (0,0)	0 (0,0)		
Level of education university*				0,8
undergraduate	09 (47,4)	10 (52,6)		
2nd cycle	16 (44,4)	20 (55,6)		
Smoking Narguile and cigarettes at the				0,1

same time				
Yes	23 (45,1)	28 (54,9)		
No	04 (25,0)	12 (75,0)		
Smoking electronic cigarettes and traditional cigarettes at the same time *				**0,03**
Yes	12 (75,0)	04 (25,0)	7,3 [1,9-28,9]	
No	09 (29,0)	22 (71,0)	.ref	
Smoking other forms of tobacco and traditional cigarettes at the same time *				**0,04**
Yes	22 (48,9)	23(51,1)	3,3 [1,02-10,3]	
No	05 (22,7)	05 (22,7)	.ref	

**: missing data ; .ref: reference categoric*

3.4 Frequency of cigarette smokers who have tried to stop smoking before

Of the 67 cigarette smokers, 43 (64.2%) had tried to quit smoking before. There was no significant difference according to sex (72.2% of men had tried to quit vs. 54.8% of women; p= 0.1). The fact of having tried to stop smoking cigarettes was not significantly associated with the perceived serious health effects (p= 0.2) of smoking. Similarly, the perceived degree to which smoking-related health problems affected smokers' lives was not significantly associated with the fact of having tried to stop smoking (p=0.9).

3.5 Student attitudes to cigarette smoking

The results of the comparison of students' attitudes to cigarette smoking according to smoking and non-smoking status are shown in Table XII.

3.5.1 Perception of the serious health effects of cigarettes

Of the 210 students, cigarette smokers and non-cigarette smokers, who answered the question measuring the degree of perception of the serious health effects of smoking, only 3.8% thought that smoking had no serious health effects at all, and 1.4% thought that it had some serious effects (Figure 17). There was no significant difference when comparing the responses of current cigarette smokers and non-cigarette smokers (6.0% of current cigarette smokers thought that smoking has no serious effects on health at all vs. 2.8% of non-cigarette smokers; p=0.2), (Table XII).

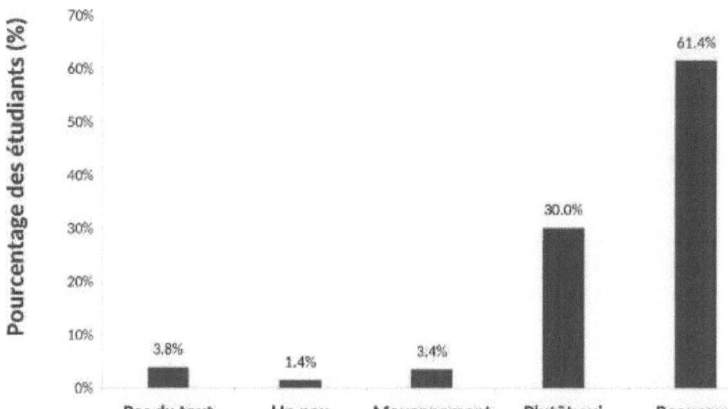

Figure 17: Degree of perception of the serious health effects of smoking among cigarette smokers and non-smokers (N=210)

3.5.2 Perceived degree to which smoking-related health problems affect life

Of the 210 students, both cigarette smokers and non-cigarette smokers, who answered the question measuring the perceived degree to which smoking-related health problems affect their lives, only 2.4% thought that smoking-related health problems do not affect smokers' lives at all, and 2.4% thought that they affect smokers' lives to a small extent (Figure 18). There was no significant difference when comparing the responses of current cigarette smokers and non-smokers (4.5% of current cigarette smokers thought that smoking does not affect smokers' lives at all vs. 1.4% of non-smokers; p=0.3), (Table XII).

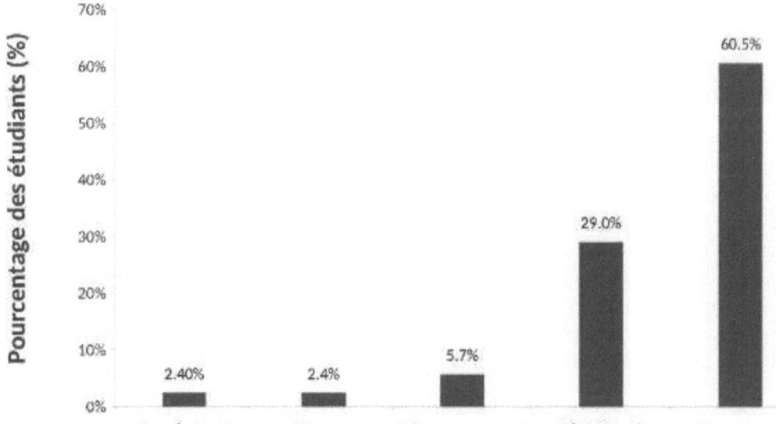

Figure 18: Smokers' and non-smokers' perception of how smoking-related health problems affect their lives (N=210)

Table XII: Comparison of students' attitudes to cigarette smoking according to smoking and non-smoking status

Student attitudes to cigarette smoking	P
Degree of perception of the **serious** health effects of	0,2

Cigarette smoking	Not at all N (% line)	Other answer N (% line)	
	smoking (N= 210)		
Cigarette smoking	**Not at all N (% line)**	**Other answer N (% line)**	
Smoker	04 (6,0)	63 (94,0)	
Non-smoking	04 (2,8)	139 (97,2)	
Cigarette smoking	Perceived degree to which smoking-related health problems **affect life** (N= 210)		0,3
	Not at all N (% line)	**Other answer N (% line)**	
Smoker	03 (4,5)	64 (95,5)	
Non-smoking	02 (1,4)	141 (98,6)	

3.5.3 Intention to start smoking cigarettes

Of the current cigarette non-smokers who answered the question (n=143) about their intention to start smoking in the next year, 134 (93.7%) had no such intention at all. While 9 students (6.3%) intended to start smoking soon, with an intensity ranging from "a little" to "moderately" (Figure 19). Intention to start smoking in the next year was not significantly associated with Narguile use (7.9% of Narguile exclusive smokers (n=38) intended to start smoking in the next year vs. 5.7% of Narguile non-smokers (n=105), p=0.7).

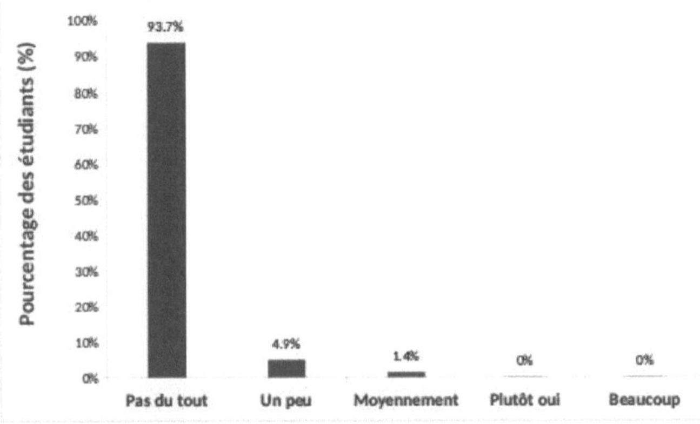

Figure 19: Non-smokers' intention to start smoking in the next year smokers (N=143)

3.5.4 Intention to stop smoking cigarettes :

Of the 67 current cigarette smokers, 94% intended to stop smoking cigarettes with an intensity ranging from "a little" to "a lot" (Figure 20). The majority (88.0%) of cigarette smokers said they were motivated to stop smoking in the next 30 days with an intensity ranging from "a little" to "a lot" (Figure 21). Similarly, the majority (89.6%) of cigarette smokers intended to reduce their smoking frequency over the next 30 days with an intensity ranging from "a little" to "a lot" (Figure 22).

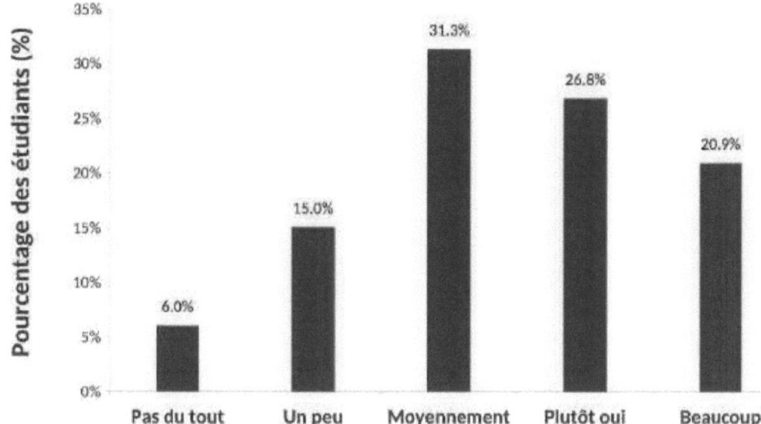

Figure 20: Current smokers' intention to quit (N=67)

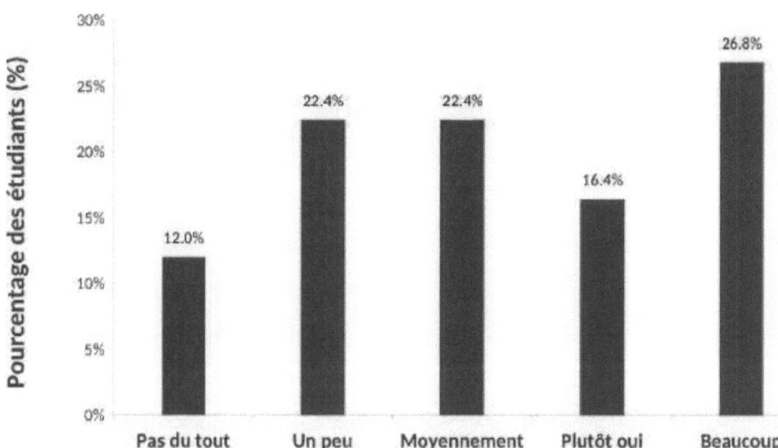

Figure 21: Level of motivation to stop smoking among current smokers (N=67)

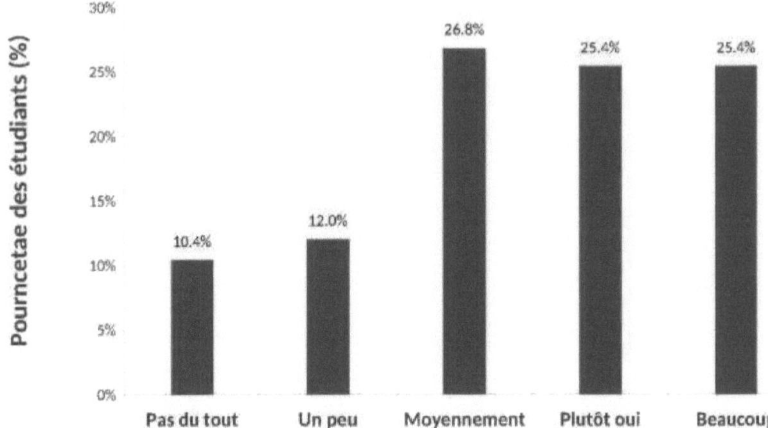

Figure 22: Current smokers' intention to reduce smoking frequency (N=67)

4. Use of other forms of tobacco

A total of 91 students (43.3%, CI95% [37.1 - 50.0]) reported having used an electronic cigarette at least once in their lifetime. Twenty-eight students (13.3%, CI95% [9.4 - 18.6]) were current e-cigarette smokers, the majority of whom (71.4%, n=20) smoked less than once a month (Figure 23).

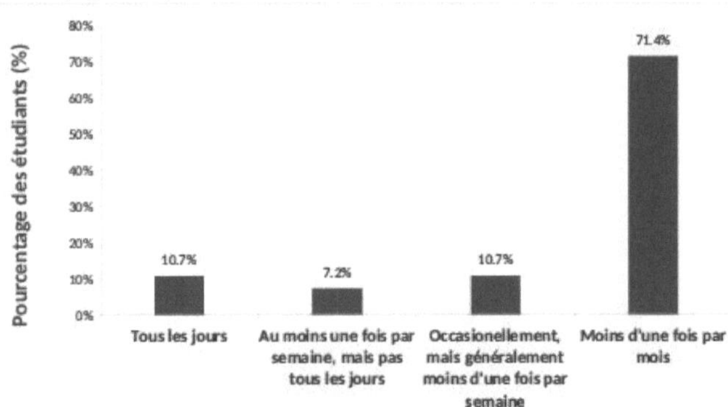

Figure 23: Breakdown of student e-cigarette smokers by frequency of use (N=28)

The frequency of use of other forms of smoking (such as cigars, *midwakh,* flavoured cigars) was 22.9% (n=48) with a 95% CI [17.6 - 28.6], of which more than half (56.3%; n= 27) smoked these forms of tobacco every day (Figure 24).

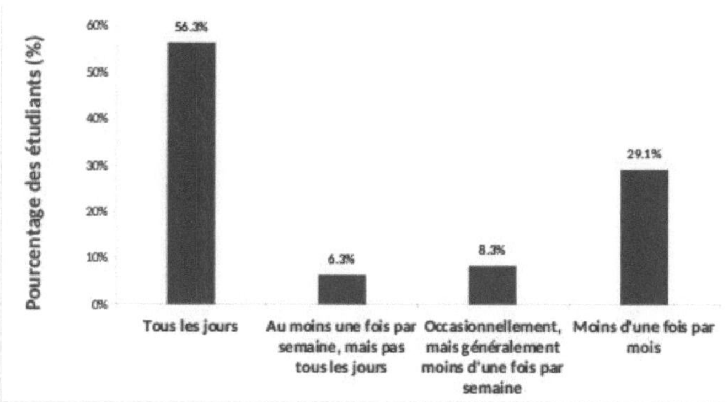

Figure 24: Breakdown of students who smoke other forms of tobacco by frequency of use (N=48)

4 DISCUSSION

The results of our study made it possible to estimate the frequency of students smoking both forms of tobacco in general. The prevalence of Narguile was very high, with more than one in 3 students (42.4%) being smokers. This prevalence was significantly higher among men ($p <10^{-3}$). The factors that were significantly associated with a higher SCTS-13 Narguile dependence score were preparing their own Narguile (p=0.04) and smoking Narguile and cigarettes at the same time (0.01). More than a fifth (21.5%) thought that Narguile was less harmful than cigarettes and 21.2% had no intention of stopping smoking Narguile. The prevalence of cigarette smoking was also high, with almost one in 3 students being smokers (31.9%), with a significantly higher prevalence among men (P<0.01).

1. Strengths and limitations of the study

One of the strong points of our study is that it is one of the few studies to have estimated the prevalence of Narguile use among young adults in Tunisia and, above all, to have assessed the degree of nicotine dependence using The Syrian Center for Tobacco Studies-13 (SCTS-13) instrument for Narguile use. This is a new instrument that was recently proposed and validated in 2020 by MM Alam et al [17] and our study was one of the few to use this score to assess the level of nicotine dependence among Narguile smokers.

We were also interested in studying the degree to which these young people perceive the evils of smoking in order to understand their attitudes and try to explain this behaviour.

In addition, we conducted our study with a sample of 210 students, which is deemed acceptable for interpreting the results with good power and precision.

However, like all scientific work, our study has certain limitations. The method used to collect the data was based on voluntary participation and did not allow us to recruit a representative sample of students, which could constitute a selection bias.

2. Discussion of results

2.1 The use of Narguile

In our study, more than a third of the students were Narguile smokers (42.4%), which represents a high prevalence.

According to a systematic review of the literature published in 2018, studying the prevalence and trends in Narguile use in 68 countries around the world, the prevalence was highest among Eastern Mediterranean countries, with prevalences of up to 37.2% among young Lebanese [4].

In another study carried out in three countries in the Eastern Mediterranean region in 2016, involving Egypt, Jordan and Palestine, the proportion of Narguile smokers was 73.8% in Egypt, 68.4% in Jordan and 63.2% in Palestine. These prevalences were very high and exceeded those found in our study [18]. Similarly, according to the results of a study carried out in Qatar in 2022, which measured the prevalence of Narguile smoking among university students, Narguile was the most commonly consumed tobacco product with a prevalence of 70.6% [19], which represented an alarming frequency and exceeded that found in our study.

Other studies carried out in 2019 and 2020 among university students in Saudi Arabia found smoking prevalences in Narguile to be slightly lower than ours, at 22.8% in 2019 and 34% in 2020 [20,21].

In another study carried out in the United Arab Emirates in 2018, which looked at knowledge, beliefs and psychosocial predictors of smoking in Narguile, the prevalence of smoking in Narguile was 38.9% and 44.9% said they had tried Narguile at least once [22].

In the western world and in Europe, several studies have been carried out to investigate smoking among young people. In a multicentre cross-sectional study carried out in Germany and Hungary in 2018, data on various aspects of health behaviour were collected from medical students. The prevalence of smoking was 18.0%, and the prevalence of Narguile use was 4.8% [23].

In the UK, a study was carried out in 6 British universities on 2217 students, using an online questionnaire, in 2015. The prevalence of Narguile smokers was 14.3% [24].

This high prevalence of Narguile smoking in Arab and Oriental countries can be explained by revolution and changing social norms, with increasing acceptability of this form of smoking. Narguile has thus become anchored in the social and traditional culture of many Arab and Oriental countries, encouraging its regular consumption. In addition, Narguile is often easily accessible in cafés and social venues, representing convivial places that encourage group consumption and contribute to its growing popularity.

Similarly, aggressive advertising and marketing can influence young people to start smoking Narguile, amplifying its prevalence. A Nigerian study was carried out in 2022 among students to investigate the moderating role of social media in the normalisation of Narguile. This study showed that the relationship between intention and impulsivity to smoke Narguile was stronger among young people who were heavily exposed to social media messages about smoking tobacco. This particular result suggests that social media messages encouraging Narguile use may increase the desire to smoke among young people [25].

In addition, the low risk perception or even the erroneous perception that Narguile is less harmful than cigarettes may also encourage its use among young people [22,26-28].

These results were consistent with those found in a study carried out in the United Arab Emirates in 2018. The study of factors associated with Narguile dependence showed a significant positive relationship between dependence, pleasure, social interaction, habit and parental smoking behaviour. The same study highlighted social interaction as one of the main factors influencing smoking behaviour in Narguile. Students tended to smoke Narguile when they were involved in social interactions in cafeterias and other places. Indeed, in most Arab countries, Narguile smoking is not stigmatised and is considered more acceptable than cigarette smoking [22].

These results were also found in a Jordanian study carried out in 2021 [29]. The students who took part in this study considered that smoking Narguile was not only considered to be socially accepted, but also to be an important and essential part of their social gathering activities. The overall acceptability of Narguile may have been achieved because of the growing popularity of this behaviour in Jordan. Narguile was on the menu of almost every restaurant in Jordan. As indicated by 35.4% of the Narguile smokers in this study, public places were the main places where Narguile was smoked.

Furthermore, at national level, the main studies carried out on smoking in Tunisia were the national "Tunisian Health Examination Survey-2016" [30], the national "Global Youth Tobacco Survey" (GYTS Survey Tunisia 2017)[31] and the latest survey, the MedSPAD III "Mediterranean School Project on Alcohol and Other Drugs" in 2021[32]. The main results of these surveys are summarised in Table XIII.

According to the national survey 'Tunisian Health Examination Survey-2016', the overall prevalence of Narguile use among the population aged over 15 was very low at 1.6% (3.1% among men vs 0.2% among women) (Table I). In the two other surveys conducted among young people, the prevalence was 7.2% (GYTS 2017) and 19.9% (MEDSAPD 2021) (Table XIII).

These low prevalences, compared with our results, can be explained by the fact that different age groups were studied in these studies compared with ours. In the GYTS and MEDSPAD studies, the population studied was younger, aged from 13 to a maximum of

18, whereas in our study, the population was aged from 18 to 34. In addition, the mode of data collection was different, with a face-to-face self-administered questionnaire in these two studies whereas the questionnaire was online in our study. This could minimise self-reporting bias as the participant feels more secure and comfortable answering online than face-to-face.

Table XIII: Main surveys on smoking prevalence in Tunisia

	National survey "Tunisian Health Examination Survey - 2016" THES 2016	**MedSPAD III survey "Mediterranean School Project on Alcohol and Other Drugs" 2021**	**National survey on smoking among young people in state schools (GYTS Survey Tunisia 2017)**
Prevalence* of smoking in percentage	Population aged 15 is 30 years old: **25,2**	**	Population aged 13 is 15 years old: **11,7**
Prevalence* of smoking by gender as a percentage	Men Women **47, 82,2**	**	Men Women **19, 24,6**
Use of cigarettes in percentage	In the population aged 15 and over more : **22,3**	Population aged 16 is 18 years old: **24,8**	Population aged 13 is 15 years old: **7,8**
Cigarette use by sex in percentage	Men Women **43, 32,0**	Men Women **41, 114,1**	Men Women **14, 41,6**
Use of narguile in percent	In the population aged 15 and over **1,6**	Population aged 16 is 18 years old: **19,9**	Population aged 13 is 15 years old: **7,2**
Oil consumption by sex in percentage	Men Women **3, 10,2**	Men Women **36, 69,3**	Men Women **132,8**

*Prevalence at least once in a lifetime

**No data

Looking at the prevalence of Narguile use by gender, according to the results of our study, male gender was significantly associated with Narguile use (60.5% in men vs. 31.0% in women; OR=3.4; p <10').^{3}

According to a study carried out in Lebanon in 2022, which included 1,117 students selected from several of the country's universities. Narguile was significantly more frequent among men (40.3% versus 29.8%; p<0.001). At the age of 11, males used Narguile significantly more than females (6.0% versus 2.2%; p<0.001) [33].

This male dominance of Narguile use is partly explained by social norms in Arab countries and the Eastern Mediterranean region, which often favour Narguile use among men and see it as a socially accepted and valued activity for strengthening social bonds [34]. This could also be explained by easier access to cafes and other social places where Narguile is available, and by the fact that they spent free time with their peers without the restrictions and surveillance experienced by women more than men. In addition, the men felt that smoking could contribute to the masculine image and perception of maturity among their peers. In addition, the social stigma of a woman smoking Narguile could explain the low prevalence of smoking among women. Moreover, the social pressure exerted on women to maintain an Islamic image that conforms to cultural norms may actually influence their behavioural choices, y including

smoking, in order to preserve their reputation and marriage prospects [33].
In a study carried out in three Eastern Mediterranean countries, among participants aged over 18 in Lebanon (n=1680), Jordan (n=1925) and Palestine (n=1679) in 2019. The prevalence of Narguile smoking among men and women was 32.7% and 46.2% respectively in Lebanon, 13.4% and 7.8% in Jordan, and 18.0% and 7.9% in Palestine. They were most frequently observed in men in Jordan and Palestine, and most frequently in women in Lebanon [35]. And in a study conducted in Saudi Arabia in 2018, there was no significant difference in the prevalence of smoking in Narguile between male and female students (25.4% versus 19.4%; p-value=0.l). The results of this study indicated that smoking in Narguile is becoming more popular and more common among young people of both sexes [20]. This trend towards equal prevalence of Narguile consumption between the sexes was also found among Jordanian students in a study conducted in 2021. These results confirm the continuing increase in Narguile smoking habits among young women in Jordan [29].
In our study, 94.4% of student smokers felt that they were not addicted to Narguile. The mean Narguile dependence score SCTS-13 was not very high (6.7 ± 5.0) out of a maximum score of 26.
According to the results of our study, being a Narguile and cigarette smoker at the same time was significantly associated with a higher SCTS-13 total Narguile dependence score. This suggests that the concomitant consumption of Narguile and cigarettes could aggravate dependence on Narguile. Indeed, the combination of two types of smoking may increase the addictive effects, as they may act synergistically to reinforce dependence [36]. Smokers of Narguile and cigarettes may develop cross-tolerance, which means that they require higher doses of nicotine to satisfy their addiction, thereby increasing their dependence on Narguile [37]. In addition, individuals likely to smoke both Narguile and cigarettes may have personality traits or addictive behaviours with consumption patterns that make them more prone to tobacco dependence in general [38,39].
Similarly, self-preparation of Narguile was significantly associated with a higher SCTS-13 total Narguile dependence score. This suggests that direct involvement in the preparation of Narguile could reinforce dependence on this practice as well as being one of the aspects of dependence.
Looking at the attitudes of the students in our study towards Narguile use, almost a third of the students thought that Narguile use is less addictive than cigarettes. In a study of Narguile smokers in five neighbouring Eastern Mediterranean countries, 44% of smokers thought that Narguile smoking was less addictive than cigarettes [40]. In another Jordanian study carried out in 2020, 29% thought that it was less addictive than cigarettes, which is in line with our results [29].
More than a fifth of the students in our study either thought that using Narguile was less harmful than smoking cigarettes or were unaware of this information. The frequency of Narguile smokers who thought that Narguile was less harmful to health than cigarettes was significantly higher than that of Narguile non-smokers. And more than a fifth of the students thought that Narguile use had little or no serious effect on health.
Our results were similar to those found in a Jordanian study carried out in 2020 among 966 university students, in which 16% of participants agreed that smoking Narguile was less harmful to health compared with cigarettes [29]. Similarly, in a cross-sectional study carried out in Saudi Arabia on the perceived harmfulness of Narguile, 38.4% of participants replied that Narguile was less harmful [21].
According to the same study, the low perception of the risks associated with Narguile was seven times higher among Narguile smokers [21]. Despite the scientific evidence of

the harmful effects and dependence associated with Narguile, it is often perceived as a safe alternative to cigarettes because of false beliefs about its safety. Studies show that this misperception stems from the idea that smoking Narguile is less harmful than cigarettes, which is unfounded. The reality is that Narguile exposes users to similar or even greater risks of cardiovascular and respiratory disease and cancer, due to the toxic smoke inhaled. A single session of Narguile smoking has been shown to be associated with more than 100 times the volume of smoke inhaled and higher levels of nicotine, tar and carbon monoxide than a single cigarette, contrary to the misconception that the water used in the pipe absorbs the toxic elements [41]. This false perception contributes to its widespread use, especially among young people, despite warnings from health authorities [42,43].

According to the results of our study, more than a fifth of students intended to start using Narguile in the near future. This is an alarming finding, as it could lead to a significant increase in the prevalence of this practice, exacerbating an already worrying problem of heavy use of Narguile among young people. Faced with this growing threat, it is imperative that urgent and immediate preventive measures be taken to counter the spread of Narguile use among young people. These measures should be based on effective public health and awareness-raising strategies.

On the other hand, of the current Narguile smokers in our study, more than one-fifth (21.2%) had no intention at all of stopping smoking Narguile. These results highlight a major challenge in the fight against Narguile consumption among young people, with a large proportion of Narguile smokers resistant to giving up this habit. Similarly, the intention to quit was significantly lower among smokers who thought that Narguile use had no serious health effects at all, and among those who thought that the health problems associated with Narguile use did not affect a smoker's life at all. This highlights the importance of targeted interventions aimed at making users aware of the risks associated with Narguile and promoting smoking cessation programmes specific to this practice.

Among the interventions that had proved effective in raising public awareness of the health risks of smoking were health warning labels on tobacco packets. In this context, a cross-sectional study was conducted in 2016 in three Eastern Mediterranean countries: Egypt, Jordan and Palestine [18]. Its objective was to study the association between health entertainment labels and motivation to quit smoking Narguile among university students who smoke. The health entertainment labels consisted of nine text messages and four messages that included both text and images. The pictorial health entertainment label "Protect your children: Don't let them be exposed to Narguile smoke" was the most likely to motivate current smokers to quit. These results were in line with a recent international expert consensus, where labels relating to the harmful effects of Narguile on newborns were identified as being among the most effective in communicating the risks associated with tobacco smoking [18].

A systematic review of smoking prevention and control interventions in Narguile was carried out in 2021. The study selected 27 interventions and grouped them into four main categories, including prevention and control interventions, and the adoption and implementation of legislation and policies to control Narguile at national and international levels. The review concluded that interventions in schools, in particularly among adolescents, may yield promising results in preventing and controlling the use of narcotics and reducing the effects of this major social and health crisis worldwide [44].

2.2 Cigarette smoking

In our study, the prevalence of cigarette smoking was 31.9% (CI_{95} % [25.7 - 38.6]).

This prevalence was 22.3% in subjects aged 15 and over, according to the results of the Tunisian national THES 2016 survey [30] (table XIII).
According to the results of the GYTS 2017 study, 7.8% of students aged 13 to 15 in Tunisia smoke cigarettes [31]. Among students aged 16 to 18, almost a quarter were cigarette smokers, according to the results of MEDSPAD 2021 [32] (table XIII).
According to estimates in the WHO's 2019 report on smoking worldwide, Tunisia is among the countries with the highest prevalence of smoking (all forms) in the Eastern Mediterranean and Africa [45].
According to the results of our study, there was a significant difference according to sex. Male sex was significantly associated with cigarette smoking (44.4% of smokers were male compared with only 24% female; P<0.01, OR= 2.5). These results were also observed in the THES 2016, GYTS 2017 and MEDSPAD 2021 surveys (table XIII). This is mainly explained by the social context of smoking in Tunisia. Indeed, as elsewhere in the Middle East and North Africa, the social acceptability of smoking in all its forms among men remains a factor encouraging this scourge among young men, as already discussed above.
In a Saudi study of 895 college students in 2022, male students were 7 times more likely to be current or former smokers than females. The study explained this predilection for smoking among male students by saying that it could be justified by the fact that male smokers tended to encourage their friends to smoke in order to have activities together. They therefore spent a lot of time smoking together in cafés and other public places. In contrast, women tended to be more cautious and concerned about their health [46]. Furthermore, according to a metanalysis also carried out in Saudi Arabia in 2018 among Saudi students. Male students showed a prevalence of 26%, while among Saudi female students, the prevalence was 5%. One of the factors explaining these results was the fact that female smokers could not honestly declare their smoking status, for fear of being rejected by society. Indeed, such behaviour, particularly among women in Saudi Arabia, is considered destructive of societal values [47].
When we studied the level of nicotine dependence among cigarette smokers in our study, 40.3% were dependent. The mean Fagerstrom score was 2.6 ± 2.2.
In a Saudi study carried out in 2022 among 430 dental students. The level of nicotine dependence was assessed using the Fagerstrom test, and 50% were moderately to strongly dependent on nicotine [48].
Another study to assess the prevalence of smoking habits among students at King Khalid University in Saudi Arabia in 2022 showed that 67% had a "moderate" to "high" dependence score [49].
In our study, the factors significantly associated with nicotine dependence were male gender, Гаде > 24 years and being a smoker of several forms of smoking at the same time (electronic cigarette, cigar, Midwakh...). Indeed, biological differences between the sexes can influence the way nicotine is metabolised in the body, thus affecting the level of dependence [50]. Also, the length of exposure to smoking could further reinforce the physical and psychological dependence on nicotine, which explains the higher level of dependence in older students [51,52]. In addition, simultaneous consumption of different forms of tobacco exposes the body to increased levels of nicotine, thereby reinforcing dependence. This may also reinforce the reward and dependence mechanisms in the brain, leading to more pronounced addiction [53].
When the students' attitudes towards cigarette smoking were studied, the majority felt that smoking had serious effects on the health of smokers. There was no significant difference when comparing the responses of current cigarette smokers and non-

smokers. Despite a good level of knowledge about its harmful effects on health, the prevalence of cigarette smoking remains high. In this respect, a Polish study carried out in 2018 among schoolchildren and students throughout the country. The research showed that young people were very aware of the harmful effects of smoking. Over 90% of smokers agreed that smoking cigarettes is bad for their health, and 80.5% thought that passive smoking had a negative effect on their health. Despite this, the prevalence of smoking was 13.7% among pupils and 20.5% among students [54].

This could be explained by several factors, such as social pressure and peer influence. Young people are often influenced by their peers and their social environment, which can encourage smoking despite knowledge of the health risks [55]. The search for immediate pleasure may also play a role. Young people may be attracted by the euphoric and stimulating effects of nicotine, seeking immediate pleasure without considering the long-term consequences [56]. Similarly, excessive advertising and marketing, often targeted at young people, create an attraction to smoking despite knowledge of the risks [57]. These factors contribute to maintaining a high prevalence of smoking among young people, even in the presence of a good understanding of the health risks.

In our study, among non-smokers, the intention to start smoking in the next year was 6.3%.

In the national survey on smoking among young people attending public colleges (GYTS Survey Tunisia 2017), the likelihood of being a smoker in the future was 9.5% (12.5% among boys vs. 7.7% among girls). Comparing these results with our study, these smoking initiation rates were higher than those found in our study [31].

In fact, the intention to start smoking is higher in adolescents than in older adults for a number of reasons. Adolescents are particularly sensitive to peer influences and social pressure, which may lead them to experiment with smoking in order to fit in socially or to imitate their friends who smoke. Adolescence is a period of identity-seeking and experimentation. Some adolescents may see smoking as a way of rebelling, feeling more grown-up or coping with stress [58]. Similarly, adolescents' vulnerability to tobacco industry marketing, which aims to glamourise cigarette smoking and create an appeal for smoking, plays an important role at initiation [59]. According to the National Survey on Tobacco Use among Young People in Public Colleges (GYTS Survey Tunisia 2017), with regard to tobacco advertising, among students who had watched television or videos in the previous months, 79.4% had reported seeing tobacco advertising messages. Similarly, 43.7% of students had been exposed to pro-tobacco advertising. Also in the context of exposure to pro-tobacco messages, 25.7% of students reported having worn clothing or objects with pro-tobacco advertising, and 12.7% said they were in possession of this type of clothing. As for the possible use of tobacco company representatives to offer gifts with pro-tobacco advertising, this was reported by 5.6% of students [31].

Similarly, the brain is in full development during adolescence, which makes them more likely to take risks and give in to impulses, y including that of experimenting with tobacco [60]. These factors contribute to a higher intention to initiate cigarette smoking in adolescents than in older adults.

Our study also showed that 94% of smokers intended to stop smoking cigarettes. The majority said they were motivated to stop smoking in the next 30 days. Similarly, the majority of cigarette smokers intended to reduce their smoking frequency over the next 30 days.

According to the GYTS 2017 survey, 74.0% of smokers said they wanted to stop smoking. However, only 17.7% of these students had sought help to stop smoking,

either through a programme or a health professional. According to the survey, a quarter (25.3%) of students thought it was difficult to quit smoking once they had started [31].
The contradiction between the desire to stop smoking declared by the majority of students and their persistence in smoking can be explained by several factors. Nicotine dependence is one of these factors. Nicotine addiction creates physical and psychological dependence, making it difficult to stop smoking despite the desire and motivation to do so [61]. Students may also be influenced by those around them, particularly other smokers, which makes it more difficult to quit. Some students may use smoking as a way of coping with stress, anxiety or academic pressures, which complicates their efforts to stop smoking [62].
It is therefore crucial to support these students in their efforts to stop smoking by offering them appropriate psychological and medical support. Effective interventions include personalised advice, smoking cessation programmes and regular follow-up to maximise the chances of success [63].
Furthermore, according to our study, 13.3% of students were current e-cigarette smokers, 71.1% of whom smoked less than once a month.
According to the National Survey on Smoking by Young People in State Colleges (GYTS Survey Tunisia 2017), e-cigarette use in the last 30 days was 4.9%, with a higher prevalence among boys than girls (7.4% vs. 2.3%) [31].
In the MedSPAD 2021 survey, the prevalence of use of electronic cigarettes, at least once in their lives, was reported by a quarter (25.3%) of secondary school students. Use of these devices was reported by 17.2% of secondary school students during the previous year and by 8.2% of secondary school students during the previous month [32].
According to the WHO, the use of electronic cigarettes is becoming increasingly popular among adolescents, with around a third of them having tried this device [64].
It has been shown that there is a significant and positive association between the use of electronic cigarettes and smoking among young people, indicating that this type of cigarette could encourage smoking among adolescents [65].
This trend of increasingly popular use of e-cigarettes among young people could be due in part to marketing aimed at young people. E-cigarette manufacturers often use aggressive, targeted marketing strategies to attract young people, particularly through social networks and online advertising, creating a new market for their products. In addition, e-cigarettes offer a variety of attractive flavours, such as fruit or sweets, which are particularly appealing to young people. Similarly, the perceived safety of this type of product could encourage them to use it more readily. In fact, some young people wrongly believe that electronic cigarettes are less harmful than traditional cigarettes, which encourages them to try them [66]. Similarly, the ease of access to e-cigarettes, including online, and the lack of strict regulations on their sale contribute to their popularity among young people [67].
This is a growing global problem linked to the use of e-cigarettes among young people, underlining the need for preventive measures and awareness-raising about the potential dangers of e-cigarettes, particularly in terms of nicotine dependence and adverse health effects, to reduce this trend and protect the health of young people. In addition, strict regulations on the marketing and sale of electronic cigarettes can help to reduce their accessibility to young people.

3. Tobacco control in the world and in Tunisia

WHO tobacco control is conducted mainly through the WHO Framework Convention on Tobacco Control (WHO FCTC) [68]. This international treaty was adopted in 2003 and came into force in 2005. To date, more than 180 parties have signed the Convention, making it one of the most widely accepted public health treaties in the world. It aims to promote effective policies to reduce tobacco consumption and limit exposure to second-hand smoke. The main objective of this convention is to protect present and future generations from the dangers of tobacco by putting in place prevention and control measures. It recommends measures such as a ban on tobacco advertising, promotion and sponsorship, and the introduction of smoke-free zones in public places. The FCTC commits signatory countries to cooperate in combating the illicit trade in tobacco products, to promote tax policies to discourage consumption, and to support smoking cessation programmes.

Within the framework of the FCTC, the MPOWER strategy [69], promoted by the WHO, offers a global framework for tobacco control by providing clear guidelines on the priority actions to be taken to reduce tobacco consumption and its harmful effects on public health. This strategy proposes six measures with a good cost-effectiveness ratio:

- **Monitoring:** This involves monitoring tobacco consumption and prevention policies, collecting data to assess the scale of the problem and the effectiveness of interventions.
- **Protection:** This component involves protecting people from tobacco smoke by introducing policies to create smoke-free public and work spaces, as well as restrictions on tobacco advertising, promotion and sponsorship.
- **Offering help:** Offering smokers help to stop smoking is a crucial aspect of tobacco control. The aim is to provide smoking cessation services and raise awareness of their accessibility.
- **The warning:** This component involves the use of striking health warnings on cigarette packets to inform consumers of the dangers of smoking.

Standards: Drawing up and applying laws to regulate tobacco advertising, promotion and sponsorship, as well as the packaging and labelling of tobacco products.

Resources: Allocate financial resources to support the implementation of smoke-free policies and the provision of health services for smokers.

It has been shown that if these measures were fully implemented and adhered to, the expected prevalence of smoking in the countries of the Eastern Mediterranean Region could fall by almost 10% by 2030 [69].

In accordance with the guidelines of the WHO Framework Convention on Tobacco Control, which was ratified by Tunisia in 2010 [70], Tunisia has implemented a number of measures to combat smoking, in particular:

Tobacco control legislation: Adoption of laws regulating direct and indirect advertising and tobacco consumption in public places, such as Law 98-17 of 1998 on tobacco control and Decree 2009-2611 of 2009 [71,72].

With a ban on smoking in public places, public transport and workplaces to protect non-smokers from exposure to second-hand smoke.

The last regulation in 2014 required warning labels to occupy at least 30% of tobacco packets [73].

- **Awareness and health promotion campaigns:** Promoting healthy lifestyles and encouraging people to adopt non-smoking behaviour. With campaigns to raise public awareness of the dangers of smoking, emphasising the health risks and benefits of quitting [74].
- **Smoking cessation support services:** Setting up smoking cessation support services, y including tobaccology consultations in several university hospitals.
- **Price and tax increases :** Increasing tobacco taxes to discourage consumption and reduce the financial accessibility of tobacco products [75].

4. Recommendations and outlook

Tobacco control in Tunisia is a major public health issue, aimed at reducing the prevalence of smoking and its harmful consequences for the population. A number of recommendations and prospects can be envisaged to strengthen this fight:

J **Full implementation of the WHO Framework Convention on Tobacco Control (FCTC):** Tunisia must continue to implement the provisions of the FCTC, y including the adoption of effective tobacco control policies and the promotion of awareness of the dangers of smoking.

J **Reinforcing regimentation policies:** It is essential to adopt and enforce strict tobacco regimentation policies, such as banning smoking in public places, increasing tobacco taxes and banning tobacco advertising.

J **Awareness-raising and education:** Continue to raise awareness of the dangers of tobacco and promote healthy lifestyles, particularly among young people. Include educational programmes in schools to prevent young people from taking up smoking.

J **Integrating tobacco control interventions into the healthcare system :** It is crucial to integrate tobacco control interventions into the healthcare system, in particular by providing more smoking cessation services, ensuring the availability of nicotine substitutes to facilitate smoking cessation and training healthcare professionals in the management of patients who smoke.

J **Monitoring and research:** Strengthen tobacco monitoring to assess the effectiveness of tobacco control policies and interventions, as well as research into smoking trends.

To combat the growth of smoking in Narguile in Tunisia, here are a few recommendations:

J **Education and awareness:** set up awareness campaigns to inform the public, particularly young people, about the health risks associated with smoking in Narguile, which are still poorly understood by most young people. Education about these dangers and the benefits of quitting smoking in Narguile can help to change young people's attitudes and behaviour.

J **Regiementation:** create a specific public regiementation for the sale and use of narguile, for example by restricting young people's access to cafés and places where narguile is consumed, and by imposing health warnings on products.

J **Access to smoking cessation services:** support smoking cessation services with specific measures for the use of Narguile to support those who wish to stop smoking Narguile like cigarettes.

J **Surveillance and Research:** strengthen the surveillance of smoking in Narguile through regular epidemiological studies to monitor trends and assess the effectiveness of prevention measures.

For measures specific to university students, we could add to those mentioned above, the creation of smoke-free areas within universities to discourage consumption, promote a healthy environment and reduce exposure to passive smoking. In addition, smoking cessation support programmes should be set up specifically for university students. These programmes could offer personalised support, advice on quitting methods, support group sessions and accessible online resources. Similarly, encourage the promotion of healthy alternatives to smoking, such as physical exercise, meditation and other relaxing activities. Organising events and activities that highlight these alternatives can help to distract students from smoking.

Persuasive posters can also play a significant role in the fight against smoking among university students. In fact, the existence of these posters in the university environment could offer several advantages:

- **Raising awareness:** posters can inform students about the dangers of smoking and Narguile, highlighting the health risks and social consequences of these addictions.

- **Influencing behaviour:** persuasive messages can influence students' attitudes and behaviour towards smoking, by providing them with convincing arguments for quitting or not starting.
- **Accessibility:** posters placed in strategic locations in universities are easily accessible to students, increasing their exposure to anti-smoking messages.
- **Group effect:** posters can also influence the behaviour of peers, as students are likely to be influenced by the social norms and attitudes of their peers.

By combining persuasive posters with other anti-smoking strategies, such as awareness campaigns and smoke-free environments, universities can effectively help to reduce the prevalence of smoking in all its forms among their students.

Following the results of our study, which was conducted on a non-representative sample of university students, there are several perspectives for future work that could be explored. Carry out studies on a representative sample of university students, including higher education establishments on a national scale. The results obtained will be more generalizable to the entire student population. This will provide a more accurate estimate of the prevalence of smoking in all its forms, including cigarettes and Narguile, among young adults attending higher education establishments across the country. Face-to-face self-administered questionnaires can provide better quality data than online surveys and help to minimise non-response rates and ensure that questionnaires are completed correctly.

Similarly, it would be interesting to explore in more detail the risk factors associated with the prevalence of smoking, especially in Narguile among university students. These could include cultural and psychological factors, academic stress, social pressures, factors relating to access to tobacco products, and so on. An in-depth analysis of these factors could help to develop more targeted prevention and intervention strategies.

In addition to quantitative data, in-depth qualitative studies could be carried out. This could involve individual interviews or focus groups to explore in depth students' perceptions, attitudes and experiences of smoking. A qualitative approach could help to understand the underlying motivations behind the behaviours observed, the triggers for smoking initiation, and the associated addiction mechanisms. All this could help to identify more effective ways of intervening.

These studies could contribute to a better understanding of the phenomenon of smoking among young adults and to the development of effective strategies to prevent and reduce this scourge.

Finally, the alarming prevalence of smoking among young university students, including cigarette and Narguile consumption, constitutes a major public health problem that requires immediate intervention. Specifically tailored prevention and awareness-raising initiatives must be put in place, and existing anti-smoking policies must be strengthened, in order to reverse this worrying trend and encourage healthier behaviour among young Tunisians. A comprehensive approach, involving the authorities, higher education establishments, civil society and the media, is essential if this public health challenge is to be tackled effectively.

5 CONCLUSIONS

Smoking is a major public health issue worldwide because of its high prevalence, its harmful effects on health and its heavy economic impact. Its incidence has increased alarmingly over the last two decades, especially in the Eastern Mediterranean region. Tunisia has not been spared this serious scourge. Despite the fact that young adults have been shown to be the group most at risk of experimenting with (initiation to) and regularly consuming Narguile, few Tunisian studies have examined the use, attitudes and dependence of this population.

Thus, the main objective of this study was to estimate the prevalence of smoking in its two main forms, i.e. cigarette and Narguile use, among university students in Tunisia. Secondly, our objectives were to describe the degree of perception of harm and the intention to stop among users of these two forms of smoking. And also to determine the level of dependence and the factors associated with it.

This was a descriptive cross-sectional survey of students at the University of Tunis El Manar. This study was conducted exclusively online between July 2021 and January 2022. We included in our study students aged between 18 and 34, living in Tunisia (for at least 5 years), with an active e-mail address belonging to the University of Tunis El Manar. Students who refused to give their informed consent before answering the questionnaire were excluded from the study.

The questionnaire consisted of four parts. One part concerned socio-demographic data (age, sex, educational level, marital status). Two other parts concerned the use of Narguile and cigarettes (frequency of use, intention to start and stop, degree of perception of harm, dependence). The level of dependence on Narguile was assessed by The Syrian Center for Tobacco Studies-13 (SCTS-13) score, which comprised 13 items with three possible responses for each item: 'False', 'Somewhat true' or 'True'. This score can vary between 0 and 26. The higher the score, the greater the degree of nicotine dependence. The level of dependence on cigarettes was assessed using the Fagerstrom score. This score is made up of 6 items. The Fagerstrom score varies between 0 and 10. A subject is classified as being weakly, moderately or strongly dependent if the score is equal to or exceeds 3 points. A final part of the questionnaire concerns other forms of tobacco consumption, such as electronic cigarettes.

A total of 210 students were included in the study, with an average age of 21.5 ± 2.3 years and a sex ratio (M/F)= 0.63. In our study, more than a third of the students were Narguile smokers (42.4%), which represents a high prevalence. According to estimates in the WHO's 2019 report on smoking (all forms) worldwide, Tunisia is among the countries with the highest prevalence of smoking among the countries of the Eastern Mediterranean and Africa. This prevalence was also quite high in other Eastern Mediterranean countries. This could be explained by revolution and changing social norms with increasing acceptability of this form of smoking in the East. Similarly, aggressive advertising and marketing may influence young people to start smoking in Narguile, amplifying its prevalence. This prevalence was significantly higher among men ($p < 10^{-3}$). This was observed in several other studies in Eastern Mediterranean countries. This male predominance of Narguile use is partly explained by social norms in Arab countries and the Eastern Mediterranean region, which often favour Narguile use among men and consider it to be a socially accepted and valued activity for strengthening social ties. In addition, the social pressure exerted on women to maintain an Islamic image that conforms to cultural norms may well influence their behavioural choices, y including smoking, in order to preserve their reputation and marriage prospects. The mean Narguile dependence score SCTS-13 was not very high (6.7 ± 5.0) out of a maximum score of 26. The factors that were significantly associated with a higher SCTS-13 Narguile dependence score were the fact of preparing one's own Narguile (p=0.04) and the fact of smoking Narguile and cigarettes at the same time (0.01). This suggests that the concomitant consumption of Narguile and cigarettes could aggravate dependence on Narguile. In fact, the combination of two types of smoking may increase the addictive effects, as they may act synergistically to reinforce dependence. Almost a third of the students thought that Narguile use was less addictive than cigarettes, which is consistent with other studies in Eastern Mediterranean countries. More than a fifth of the students in our study thought that Narguile use was less harmful than cigarettes, or were unaware of this information. The low perception of the risks or even the erroneous perception that Narguile is less harmful than cigarettes may further encourage its use among young people.

More than a fifth of smokers had no intention at all of stopping smoking Narguile. This intention to quit was significantly lower among smokers with erroneous knowledge about the harms of Narguile. This underlines the importance of targeted interventions aimed at making users aware of the risks associated with Narguile and promoting smoking cessation programmes specific to this practice.

The prevalence of cigarette smoking was 31.9% (95% CI [25.7 - 38.6]). This prevalence was 22.3% among subjects aged 15 and over, according to the results of the Tunisian national THES 2016 survey. Male sex was significantly associated with cigarette smoking (P<0.01). These results were also observed in the THES 2016, GYTS 2017 and MEDSPAD 2021 surveys. This is mainly explained by the social context of smoking in Tunisia. Indeed, as elsewhere in the Middle East and North Africa, the social acceptability of smoking in all its forms among men remains a factor encouraging this scourge among young men.

When studying students' attitudes to cigarette smoking, the majority felt that tobacco had serious effects on smokers' health. Despite a good level of knowledge about its health effects, the prevalence of cigarette smoking remains high. This could be explained by a number of factors, such as social pressure and peer influence, the search for immediate pleasurable sensations, and excessive advertising and marketing, often targeted at young people, which create an attraction to smoking despite knowledge of the risks. Our study also showed that 94% of smokers intended to stop smoking cigarettes. The majority said they were motivated to stop smoking in the next 30 days. The contradiction between the desire to stop smoking declared by the majority of students and their persistence in smoking may be explained by nicotine dependence and the influence of their entourage and peers. Some students may also use smoking as a way of coping with stress, anxiety or academic pressures, which complicates their efforts to stop smoking.

Furthermore, according to our study, 13.3% of students were current electronic cigarette smokers. According to the WHO, the use of electronic cigarettes is becoming increasingly popular among teenagers, with around a third of them having tried the device. This trend of increasingly popular use of electronic cigarettes among young people could be due in part to marketing aimed at young people. In addition, electronic cigarettes offer a variety of attractive flavours, which are particularly appealing to young people. Similarly, the perceived safety of this type of product could encourage them to use it more readily. Indeed, some young people wrongly believe that electronic cigarettes are less harmful than traditional cigarettes, which encourages them to try them.

Tobacco control by the WHO is carried out mainly through the WHO Framework Convention on Tobacco Control (FCTC). The main objective of this convention is to protect present and future generations from the dangers of tobacco by putting in place prevention and control measures. The MPOWER strategy, promoted by the WHO, offers a global framework for tobacco control by providing clear guidelines on the priority actions to be taken to reduce tobacco consumption and its harmful effects on public health. This strategy proposes six cost-effective measures (monitoring tobacco consumption, protecting people from tobacco smoke, offering help to smokers to quit, warning through the use of health warnings on tobacco packages, developing and enforcing laws to regulate tobacco advertising, promotion and sponsorship, and allocating financial resources to support the implementation of smoke-free policies).

In line with the guidelines of the WHO Framework Convention on Tobacco Control, which was ratified by Tunisia in 2010, Tunisia has implemented a number of measures to combat smoking: anti-smoking legislation, awareness-raising and health promotion campaigns, the introduction of services to help people stop smoking, and higher taxes on tobacco to discourage consumption and reduce financial access to tobacco products. Despite these efforts, the prevalence of smoking in all its forms remains high. All these measures must be maintained and further strengthened in order to reduce this scourge among young people.

To combat the growth in Narguile smoking among young people in Tunisia, it is necessary to set up awareness-raising campaigns on the health risks associated with Narguile smoking, which are still poorly understood by most young people. A specific regulation should also be created for the advertising, sale and use of Narguile. Support smoking cessation services with specific measures for Narguile use to help those who want to stop smoking Narguile. Creating smoke-free spaces in universities to discourage consumption and promote a healthy environment. As well as setting up smoking cessation support programmes specifically designed for university students and encouraging the promotion of healthy alternatives to smoking, such as physical exercise, meditation and other relaxing activities. Persuasive posters can also play a significant role in the fight against smoking among students.

Following the results of our study, which was conducted on a non-representative sample of university students, there are several perspectives for future work that could be explored. Carry out studies on a representative sample of university students, including higher education establishments on a national scale. The results obtained would be more generalisable to the student population as a whole. Similarly, it would be interesting to explore in more detail the risk factors associated with the prevalence of smoking, especially in Narguile among university students. These could include cultural factors, psychological factors, academic stress, social pressures, factors of accessibility to tobacco products, etc. An in-depth analysis of these factors could help to develop more targeted prevention and intervention strategies. A qualitative approach could help to understand the underlying motivations behind the behaviours observed, the factors triggering smoking initiation, and the associated mechanisms of dependence. These studies could contribute to a better understanding of the phenomenon of smoking among young adults and to the implementation of effective strategies to prevent and reduce this scourge.

In conclusion, the alarming prevalence of smoking among young university students, including cigarette and Narguile consumption, constitutes a major public health problem that requires immediate intervention. Specifically tailored prevention and awareness-raising initiatives must be put in place, and existing anti-smoking policies must be strengthened, in order to reverse this worrying trend and encourage healthier behaviour among young Tunisians. A comprehensive approach, involving the authorities, higher education establishments, civil society and the media, is essential if this public health challenge is to be tackled effectively.

6 REFERENCES

1. World Health Organization. WHO report on the global tobacco epidemic, 2021 addressing new and emerging products. [Online], Nov 2021 [Accessed 27 March 2024]. Available at
l'URL:https://iris.who.int/bitstream/handle/10665/343287/9789240032095-eng.pdf?sequence=l
2. Institute for Health Metrics and Evaluation. GBD Results. [Online], Dec 2021 [Accessed 27 March 2024]; [185 pages]. Available from URL: https://vizhub.healthdata.org/gbd-results
3. World Health Organization. Risk factors. [Online]. Feb 2020 [Accessed 27 March 2024]; [185 pages]. Available from: URL:
http://www.emro.who.int/fr/noncommunicable-diseases/causes/risk-factors.html
4. Jawad M, Charide R, Waziry R, Darzi A, Bailout RA, Akl EA. The prevalence and trends of waterpipe tobacco smoking: a systematic review. PLoS One. 2018 Feb;13(2):e0192191.
5. Alanazi N. Waterpipe smoking in Saudi Arabia: action plan. Tob Indue Dis. 2019 Apr;17:38.
6. Tucktuck M, Ghandour R, Abu Rmeileh NE. Waterpipe and cigarette tobacco smoking among Palestinian university students: a cross-sectional study. BMC Public Health. 2017 Jul;18(l):l.
7. Akl EA, Ward KD, Bteddini D, Khaliel R, Alexander AC, Lotfi T, et al. The allure of the waterpipe: a narrative review of factors affecting the epidemic rise in waterpipe smoking among young persons globally. Tob Control. 2015 Mar;24 Suppl 1:13-21.
8. Abu Rmeileh NE, Alkhuffash O, Kheirallah K, Mostafa A, Darawad M, Al Farsi Y, et al. Harm perceptions of waterpipe tobacco smoking among university students in five eastern mediterranean region countries: a cross-sectional study. Tob Indue Dis. 2018 May;16:20.
9. Akl EA, Jawad M, Lam WY, Co CN, Obeid R, Irani J. Motives, beliefs and attitudes towards waterpipe tobacco smoking: a systematic review. Harm Reduct J. 2013 Jul;10:12.
10. Qasim H, Alarabi AB, Alzoubi KH, Karim ZA, Alshbool FZ, Khasawneh FT. The effects of hookah/waterpipe smoking on general health and the cardiovascular system. Environ Health Prev Med. 2019 Sep;24(l):58.
11. Institut National de la Sante. La sante des Tunisiens results de l'enquete "Tunisian Health Examination Survey-2016". [On line], Feb 2019 [Accessed on 27 mars 2024];[185 pages]. Available at l'URL:
http://www.santetunisie.rns.tn/images/rapport-final-enquete2020.pdf
12. Murray CL. Global burden of 87 risk factors in 204 countries and territories, 1990-2019: a systematic analysis for the global burden of disease study 2019. Lancet. 2020 Oct;396(10258):1223-49.
13. World Health Organization. Tunisia 2010 (ages 13-15) global youth tobacco survey (GYTS) fact sheet. [Online], June 2012 [Accessed 27 March 2024]. Available at URL:
https://www.emro.who.int/images/stories/tfi/documents/gyts_fs_tun_2010.pdf7ua =1
14. World Health Organization. Waterpipe tobacco smoking & health[1] [Online], May 2015 [Accessed 27 March 2024]. Available at URL:
https://iris.who.int/bitstream/handle/10665/179523/WHO_NMH_PND_15.4_eng.pdf?sequence=l
15. Alam MM, Ward KD, Bahelah R, Kalan ME, Asfar T, Eissenberg T, et al. The Syrian center for tobacco studies-13 (SCTS-13): psychometric evaluation of a waterpipespecific nicotine dependence instrument. Drug Alcohol Depend. 2020 Oct;215:108192.
16. Heatherton TF, Kozlowski LT, Frecker RC, Fagerstrom KO. The fagerstrom test for

nicotine dependence: a revision of the fagerstrom tolerance questionnaire. Br J Addict. 1991 Sep;86(9):1119-27.
17. Masudul Alam M, Ward KD, Bahelah R, Kalan ME, Asfar T, Eissenberg T, et al. The Syrian center for tobacco studies-13 (SCTS-13): Psychometric evaluation of a waterpipe-specific nicotine dependence instrument. Drug Alcohol Depend. 2020 Oct;215:108192.
18. Farran D, Khawam G, Nakkash R, Lee J, Abu Rmeileh N, Darawad MW, et al. Association of health warning labels and motivation to quit waterpipe tobacco smoking among university students in the Eastern mediterranean region. Tob Prev Cessat. 2021 Jun;7:44.
19. Al Jayyousi GF, Kurdi R, Islam N, Alhussaini NZ, Awada S, Abdul Rahim H. Factors affecting waterpipe tobacco smoking among university students in Qatar. Subst Use Misuse. 2022 Dec;57(3):392-401.
20. Alshayban D, Joseph R. A Call for effective interventions to curb shisha tobacco smoking among university students in eastern province, Saudi Arabia: findings from a cross-sectional study. Asian Pac J Cancer Prev. 2019 Oct;20(10):2971-7.
21. Salih S, Shaban S, Athwani Z, Alyahyawi F, Alharbi S, Ageeli F, et al. Prevalence, predictors, and characteristics of waterpipe smoking among Jazan university students in Saudi Arabia: a cross-sectional study. Ann Glob Health. 2020 Jul;86(l):87.
22. Saravanan C, Attlee A, Sulaiman N. A cross sectional study on knowledge, beliefs and psychosocial predictors of shisha smoking among university students in Sharjah, United Arab emirates. Asian Pac J Cancer Prev. 2019 Mar;20(3):903-9.
23. Balogh E, Faubl N, Riemenschneider H, Balazs P, Bergmann A, Cseh K, et al. Cigarette, waterpipe and e-cigarette use among an international sample of medical students. Cross-sectional multicenter study in Germany and Hungary. BMC Public Health. 2018 May;18(l):591.
24. Jawad M, Choaie E, Brose L, Dogar O, Grant A, Jenkinson E, et al. Waterpipe tobacco use in the united kingdom: a cross-sectional study among university students and stop smoking practitioners. PLoS One. 2016 Jan;ll(l):e0146799.
25. Adu AO, Ismail N, Noor SM. Motivators of impulsivity to smoke waterpipe tobacco among Nigerian youth who smoke waterpipe tobacco: the moderating role of social media normalisation of waterpipe tobacco. BMC Public Health. 2022 May;22(l):1057.
26. Burki TK. Tobacco control in Jordan. Lancet Respir Med. 2019 May;7(5):386.
27. Almogbel YS, Aladhadh T, Alammar A, Aloraini A, Alghofaili S, Almutairi A, et al. Predictors of waterpipe smoking among university students in the Qassim region, Saudi Arabia. Tob Indue Dis. 2021 Aug;19:67.
28. Jafaralilou H, Latifi A, Khezeli M, Afshari A, Zare F. Aspects associated with waterpipe smoking in Iranian youths: a qualitative study. BMC Public Health. 2021 Sep;21(l):1633.
29. Al Sawalha NA, Almomani BA, Al Shatnawi SF, Almomani BN. Attitudes and knowledge of the harmful effects of waterpipe tobacco smoking among university students: a study from Jordan. Environ Sci Pollut Res Int. 2021 Aug;28(32):43725- 31.
30. Institut National de la Sante. Indicateurs clefs de la sante des Tunisiens results de l'enquete "Tunisian Health Examination Survey-2016". [On line], Fev 2019 [Consulte le 27 mars 2024]; [52 pages]. Consultable a l'URL:
http://www.santetunisie.rns.tn/images/thes-rapport2020.pdf
31. Hsairi M, Gzara A. Enquete nationale sur le tabagisme des jeunes scolarises dans les colleges publics (GYTS Survey Tunisia 2017). [Online], Oct 2017 [Accessed on 27 March 2024]; [62 pages]. Available at l'URL:
http://www.santetunisie.rns.tn/images/docs/anis/actualite/Lenqute-nationale-sur-

smoking-among-schoolchildren-in-public-schools.pdf
32. Aounallah Skhiri H, Ben Hammouda L, Ben Sassi L, Sinane L, Ben Salah N, Zid M, et al. Enquete MedSPAD III - Tunisie 2021 resultats de l'enquete nationale. [Online], Jan 2023 [Accessed 27 March 2024]; [28 pages]. Available from URL: http://www.santetunisie.rns.tn/images/medspad3_2023.pdf
33. Akel M, Sakr F, Fahs I, Dimassi A, Dabbous M, Ehlinger V, et al. Smoking behavior among adolescents: the lebanese experience with cigarette smoking and waterpipe use. Int J Environ Res Public Health. 2022 May;19(9):5679.
34. Nakkash RT, Khalil J, Afifi RA. The rise in narghile (shisha, hookah) waterpipe tobacco smoking: a qualitative study of perceptions of smokers and non-smokers. BMC Public Health. 2011 May;ll:315.
35. Nakkash R, Khader Y, Chalak A, Abla R, Abu Rmeileh NE, Mostafa A, et al. Prevalence of cigarette and waterpipe tobacco smoking among adults in three Eastern Mediterranean countries: a cross-sectional household survey. BMJ Open. 2022 Mar;12(3):e055201.
36. Bouquet L. Prevalence et facteurs associes a la consommation de narguile: une enquete anonyme par questionnaire chez des lyceens havrais. Etat des connaissances actuelles sur les risques sanitaires encourus [thesis: medecine], Rouen: Unirouen UFR Sante; 2019;91.
37. Malaeb D, Akel M, Sacre H, Haddad C, Obeid S, Hallit S, et al. Association between cumulative cigarette and Waterpipe smoking and symptoms of dependence in Lebanese adults. BMC Public Health. 2021 Aug;21(l):1583.
38. Abbadi A, Alnahar J, Zoghoul S, Bsoul A, Alarood S, Al Mistarehi AH, et al. Waterpipe nicotine dependence and depressive symptoms among adolescent waterpipe and dual users. J Environ Public Health. 2020 Nov;2020:2364571.
39. Bahelah R, Ward KD, Ben Taleb Z, Di Franza JR, Eissenberg T, Jaber R, et al. Determinants of progression of nicotine dependence symptoms in adolescent waterpipe smokers. Tob Control. 2019 May;28(3):254-60.
40. Abu Rmeileh NE, Alkhuffash O, Kheirallah K, Mostafa A, Darawad M, Al Farsi Y, et al. Harm perceptions of waterpipe tobacco smoking among university students in five eastern Mediterranean region countries: a cross-sectional study. Tob Indue Dis. 2018 May;16:20.
41. Primack BA, Carroll MV, Weiss PM, Shihadeh AL, Shensa A, Farley ST, et al.
Systematic review and meta-analysis of inhaled toxicants from waterpipe and cigarette smoking. Public Health Rep. 2016 Jan;131(l):76-85.
42. Adetona O, Mok S, Rajczyk J, Brinkman MC, Ferketich AK. The adverse health effects of waterpipe smoking in adolescents and young adults: a narrative review. Tob Indue Dis. 2021 Oct;19:81.
43. Maziak W, Ward KD, Afifi Soweid RA, Eissenberg T. Tobacco smoking using a waterpipe: a re-emerging strain in a global epidemic. Tob Control. 2004 Dec;13(4):327-33.
44. Babaie J, Ahmadi A, Abdollahi G, Doshmangir L. Preventing and controlling water pipe smoking: a systematic review of management interventions. BMC Public Health. 2021 Feb;21(l):344.
45. World Health Organization. WHO report on the global tobacco epidemic 2019: offer help to quit tobacco use. [Online], Jul 2019 [Accessed 27 Mar 2024]. Available from URL: https://www.who.int/publications-detail-redirect/9789241516204
46. Bin Abdulrahman KA, Alghamdi HA, Alfaleh RS, Albishri WS, Almuslamani WB, Alshakrah AM, et al. Smoking habits among college students at a public university in

Riyadh, Saudi Arabia. Int J Environ Res Public Health. 2022 Sep;19(18):11557.
47. Alotaibi SA, Alsuliman MA, Durgampudi PK. Smoking tobacco prevalence among college students in the Kingdom of Saudi Arabia: systematic review and metaanalysis. Tob Indue Dis. 2019 Apr;17:35.
48. Khanagar SB, Almansour AS, Alshanqiti HM, Alkathiri NF, Asseery MA, Altheyabi SM, et al. Cigarette smoking and nicotine dependence among dental students in Riyadh, Saudi Arabia: a cross-sectional study. Cureus. 2023 Nov;15(II):e48676.
49. Kandasamy G, Sam G, Almanasef M, Almeleebia T, Shorog E, Alshahrani AM, et al. A study on the prevalence of smoking habits among the student community in Aseer Region, Saudi Arabia. Front Public Health. 2023 Dec;II:1257131.
50. Pogun S, Yararbas G. Sex differences in nicotine action. In: Henningfield JE, London ED, Pogun S, eds. Nicotine psychopharmacology. Berlin: Springer; 2009. p. 261-91.
51. Mittal S, Komiyama M, Ozaki Y, Yamakage H, Satoh Asahara N, Wada H, et al. Impact of smoking initiation age on nicotine dependency and cardiovascular risk factors: a retrospective cohort study in Japan. Eur Heart J Open. 2023 Dec;4(I):135.
52. Li H, Zhou Y, Li S, Wang Q, Pan L, Yang X, et al. The relationship between nicotine dependence and age among current smokers. Iran J Public Health. 2015 Apr;44(4):495-500.
53. Jones DM, Guy MC, Fairman BJ, Soule E, Eissenberg T, Fagan P. Nicotine dependence among current cigarette smokers who use e-cigarettes and cannabis. Subst Use Misuse. 2023 Feb;58(5):618-28.
54. Zielihska Danch W. The prevalence of waterpipe tobacco smoking among polish youths. Arch Med Sci. 2019 May;17(3):731-8.
55. Jarallah JS, Bamgboye EA, Al Ansary LA, Kalantan KA. Predictors of smoking among male junior secondary school students in Riyadh, Saudi Arabia. Tob Control. 1996 Jan;5(I):26-9.
56. Fernandez L, Bonnet A, Teyssier MF, Apter MJ, Pedinielli JL, Sztulman H. Tabagisme et etats metamotivationnels chez des adolescents lyceens. Psychotropes. Nov 2004;10(2):19-46.
57. Burns DM. Use of media in tobacco control programs. Am J Prev Med. 1994 May;10 Suppl 3:3-7.
58. Lareyre O. P2P, une intervention de pair a pair visant a prevenir le tabagisme de lyceens professionnels: quel role de la theorie du comportement planifie dans le maintien des comportements de sante? [thesis : psychologies Montpellier : Universite Paul Valery; 2016.
59. Harvey J, Chadi N. Smoking prevention in children and adolescents: practice and policy recommendations. Paediatr Child Health. May 2016;21(4):209-21.
60. Constance J, Peretti Watel P. La cigarette du pauvre. Ethnologie franqaise. Mai 2010;40(3):535-42.
61. Prochaska JJ. Smoking cessation. [On-line], Nov 2023 [Accessed 27 March 2024]. Available at URL: https://www.msdmanuals.com/fr/professional/sujets-speciaux/consommation-de-tabac/sevrage-tabagique
62. 62. Stoebner Delbarre A, Annessi Maesano I, Slama K, Mekihan Cheinin P, Carton S. Smoking: management in students. [Online], July 2017 [Accessed 27 March 2024]. Available at URL: https://hal-lara.archives- ouvertes.fr/hal-01570684/document
63. Haute Autorite de Sante. Stop smoking and don't relapse. Dossier d'information patient. [Online], Jan 2024 [Accessed 27 March 2024]. Available at URL: https://www.has-sante.fr/jcms/c_1719733/fr/arreter-de-

smoking-and-not-quitting-patient-information-file
64. Azerbaijan National News Agency. WHO: electronic cigarettes are more popular than conventional cigarettes among teenagers. [Online]. Mar 2024 [Accessed 27 March 2024]. Available at URL: https://azertag.az/fr/xeber/oms electronic_cigarettes_are_more_popular what_are_conventional_cigarettes_among_adolescents-2976654
65. Watkins SL, Glantz SA, Chaffee BW. Association of noncigarette tobacco product use with future cigarette smoking among youth in the population assessment of tobacco and health (PATH) study, 2013-2015. JAMA Pediatr. 2018 Feb;172(2):181- 7.
66. Vicari S. Vaping polemic and authority discourse between influencers and institutional discourse on WEB 2.0. Argumentation and discourse analysis. [Online], Apr 2021 [Accessed on 27 March 2024]. Consultablea l'URL: https://journals.openedition.org/aad/5093
67. High Council for Public Health. Opinion on the benefits and risks of electronic cigarettes. [Online]. Nov 2021 [Accessed 27 March 2024]. Available at URL: https://www.hcsp.fr/Explore.cgi/AvisRapportsDomaine?clefr=1138
68. World Health Organization. WHO Framework Convention on Tobacco Control. [Online], Dec 2020 [Accessed 27 March 2024]. Available at URL: http://www.emro.who.int/fr/tobacco/fctc/convention-cadre-oms-lutte- antitabac.html
69. World Health Organization. Tobacco Free Initiative. MPOWER measures. [Online], Dec 2020 [Accessed 27 March 2024]. Available at URL: http://www.emro.who.int/fr/tfi/mpower/index.html
70. World Health Organization. WHO report on the global tobacco epidemic 2021: addressing new and emerging products. [Online], July 2021 [Accessed 27 March 2024]. Available at URL: https://www.who.int/publications-detail- redirect/9789240032095
71. Republique Tunisienne. Loi n° 98-17 du 23 fevrier 1998, relative a la prevention des mefaits du tabagisme (J.O. 27 fevrier 1998). Available in French: https://assets.tobaccocontrollaws.org/uploads/legislation/Tunisia/Tunisia-Law-No,- 98-17-native.pdf
72. Republique Tunisienne. Decret n° 2009-2611 du 14 septembre 2009, completant le decret n° 98-2248 du 16 novembre 1998 fixant les lieux affectes a l'usage collectif dans lesquels il est interdit de fumer (J.O. 18 septembre 2009). Available: https://assets.tobaccocontrollaws.org/uploads/legislation/Tunisia/Tunisia-Decree- No.-2009-2611-native.pdf
73. Harizi C, El Awa F, Ghedira H, Audera Lopez C, Fakhfakh R. Implementation of the WHO framework convention on tobacco control in Tunisia: progress and challenges. Tob Prev Cessat. 2020 Dec;6:72.
74. Tobacco Atlas. Global tobacco control information & statistics I Tobacco Atlas. [Online], Oct 2022 [Accessed 27 March 2024]. Available at URL: https://tobaccoatlas.org/
75. La Presse de Tunisie. Cigarettes: increase in retail prices. [Online]. Mar 2020 [Accessed 27 March 2024]. Available at URL: https://lapresse.tn/53172/cigarettes-augmentation-des-prix-de-vente-au-public/

7 APPENDICES

Appendix I: Online questionnaire

1. Demographics

1. Are you:
- Male
- Female
2. How old are you?
3. What is your nationality?
4. What is the highest level of education you have completed to date?
- Less than secondary school
- Lycee
- Undergraduate diploma / baccalaureate
- Diplôme d'etudes superieures / Master's degree

Field of study

5. Which of the following best describes your current relationship status? (Circle one)
- Single
- Marie/partner
- Widower
- Separes/Divorces

2.

6. Do you currently smoke cigarettes?
- I've never smoked, not even a puff - Continue to question 9
- I used to smoke but I stopped - Continue with question 9
- Every day - go to question 10
- At least once a week, but not every day - go to question 10
- Occasionally, but less than once a week -- go to question 10
- Less than once a month -- go to question 10
7. Do you intend to smoke cigarettes in the next year?
- Not at all
- A little
- Medium
- Yes
- Many
8. Have you ever tried to stop smoking?
- Yes
- No

Intention to stop smoking - Current cigarette smokers

9. Do you intend to stop turner?
- Not at all
- A little
- Medium
- Yes
- Many
10. Do you intend to cut down smoking in the next 30 days?
- Not at all
- A little
- Medium
- Yes
- Many
11. How motivated are you to stop smoking next month, in the next 30 days?
- Not at all
- A little
- Medium
- Yes
- Many

Fagerstrom for today's cigarette smokers

QuestionsAnswersPoints

15. How long after	Within 5 minutes	3

When you wake up, you smoke your first cigarette?	6-30 minutes 31-60 minutes After 60 minutes	2 1 0
16. Do you find it difficult to refrain from smoking in places where it is prohibited (e.g. churches, libraries, cinemas, etc.)?	Yes No	1 0
the 7. Which cigarette would you hate most	First thing in the morning Every other	1 0
18. How many cigarettes/day Do you smoke?	10 or less 11-20 21-30 31 or more	0 1 2 3
19. Do you smoke more frequently during the first few hours after waking than during the rest of the day.	Yes No	1 0
20. Do you smoke if you are so sick that you're in bed most of the day?	Yes No	1 0

Perceived harm (probability and severity) - for cigarette smokers and non-smokers smokers

These questions concern your beliefs about future health problems due to smoking. If you are not sure of the answer, please give us your best estimate.

22. To what extent do you think smoking can cause serious health effects?
- Not at all
- A little
- Medium
- Yes
- Many

23. To what extent do smoking-related health problems affect smokers' lives?
- Not at all
- A little
- Medium
- Yes
- Many

4 - Smoking Narguile

24. Do you smoke Narguile :

Yes

No

25. Do you currently smoke Narguile :
- Daily
- At least once a week, but not every day
- Occasionally, but less than once a week
- Less than once a month

26. At what age did you start smoking Narguile?

Please specify age if possible:

27. In your opinion, how "hooked" are you on Narguile?
- No grip
- A bit of an addict
- Very catchy

28. Do you own a Narguile?
- Yes
- No

29. Do you usually make your own Narguile?
- Yes
- No

30. Compared to cigarettes, do you think smoking Narguile is: *(smokers and non-smokers)*
- Less addictive
- Just as addictive
- More addictive
- I don't know

31. Do you think smoking Narguile is better than smoking cigarettes?
- Less harmful than cigarettes
- As harmful as cigarettes
- Less harmful than cigarettes
- I don't know

32. Have you ever tried to stop smoking Narguile?
- Yes
- No

Intention to stop -Nargu ile

33. Do you intend to stop smoking Narguile?
- Not at all
- A little
- Legerement
- Not bad
- Many

34. Do you intend to reduce smoking in Narguile over the next 30 days?
- Not at all
- A little
- Legerement
- Not bad
- Many

35. How motivated are you to stop smoking Narguile in the next 30 days?
- Not at all
- A little
- Legerement
- Not bad
- Many

Perceived harm (probability and severity) - smokers and non-smokers

These *questions ask about your beliefs about future health problems due to smoking in Narguile. If you are not sure of the answer, please give us your best estimate.*

37. To what extent do you think smoking Narguile can cause serious health effects?
- Not at all
- A little
- Legerement
- Not bad
- Many

38. How would the health problems associated with smoking in Narguile affect the life of a Narguile smoker?
- Not at all
- A little
- Legerement

- Not bad
- Many

The Syrian Center for Tobacco Studies-13 (SCTS-13)				
SCTS-1	**Most of my friends smoke Narguile**	False **(0)**	A little true **(1)**	True **(2)**
SCTS-2	**Just the sight or smell of a water pipe is enough to make me want to smoke.**	False **(0)**	A little true **(1)**	True **(2)**
SCTS-3	**Even if I was sure that Narguile wasn't good for my health, I'd still smoke just as often.**	False **(0)**	A little true **(1)**	True **(2)**
SCTS-4	**Smoking Narguile makes me**	False **(0)**	A little true **(1)**	True **(2)**

	happy			
SCTS-5	**Smoking Narguile makes me feel energised**	False **(0)**	A little true **(1)**	True **(2)**
SCTS-6	**If the cost of Narguile doubled, I'd still smoke as often as ever.**	False **(0)**	A little true **(1)**	True **(2)**
SCTS-7	**When I smoke Narguile, I feel less sad or depressed**	False **(0)**	A little true **(1)**	True **(2)**
SCTS-8	**It would be very difficult for me to be in a restaurant and not smoke Narguile.**	False **(0)**	A little true **(1)**	True **(2)**
SCTS-9	**Smoking Narguile is a good way of rewarding myself**	False **(0)**	A little true **(1)**	True **(2)**
SCTS-10	**It would be difficult for me to refuse an invitation to smoke Narguile**	False **(0)**	A little true **(1)**	True **(2)**
SCTS-11	**I usually smoke Narguile with friends or in cafes/restaurants.**	False **(0)**	A little true **(1)**	True **(2)**
SCTS-12	**If my smoking session were to be interrupted, I'd be upset.**	False **(0)**	A little true **(1)**	True **(2)**
SCTS-13	**When I smoke a water pipe, I feel less irritable, frustrated or angry.**	False **(0)**	A little true **(1)**	True **(2)**

Other smoking methods (cigarette smokers and non-smokers)

38. Do you currently smoke a cigar, a little cigar, a cigarillo, a midwakh or a flavoured cigar?
- Usually every day
- Usually at least once a week, but not every day
- Occasionally, but generally less than once a week
- Less than once a month
- Not at all

39. Have you ever used an electronic cigarette or an electronic cigarette, even just once in your whole life?

a. Yes

b. No

40. Do you currently smoke or vape an electronic cigarette or cigarette? a. Usually every day

b. Usually at least once a week, but not every day

c. Occasionally, but generally less than once a week

d. Less than once a month

e. Not at all

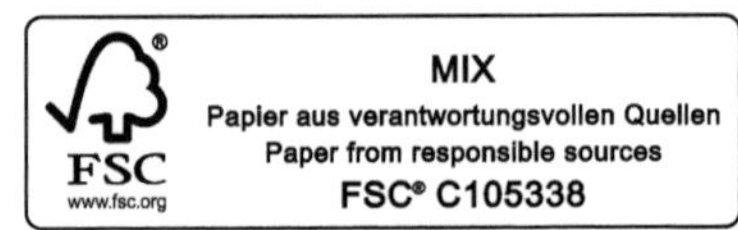

Printed by Books on Demand GmbH, Norderstedt / Germany